MW01274008

"MOTHER AND CHILD WERE SAVED"

The memoirs (1693-1740) of the Frisian midwife Catharina Schrader

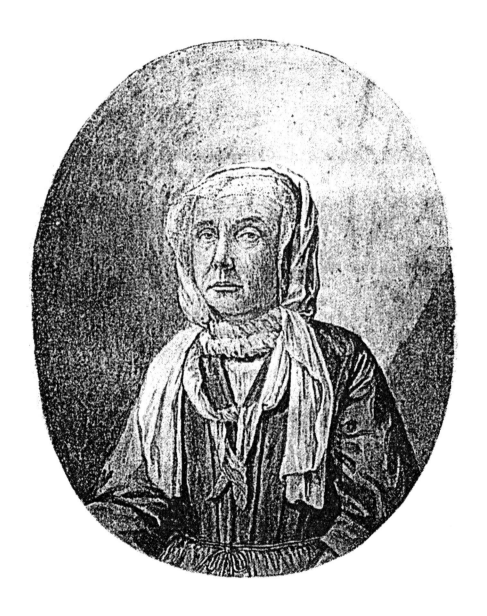

Portrait of Catharina Geertruida Schrader (1656-1746). A wash drawing by J. Folkema, 1714 (Iconographical Office, The Hague).

"MOTHER AND CHILD WERE SAVED"

The memoirs (1693-1740) of the Frisian midwife Catharina Schrader

Translated and annotated by Hilary Marland
With introductory essays
by
M.J. van Lieburg
and
G.J. Kloosterman

AMSTERDAM 1987

Nieuwe Nederlandse Bijdragen tot de Geschiedenis der Geneeskunde en der Natuurwetenschappen

No. 22

The paper on which this book is printed meets the requirements of "ISO 9706:1994, Information and documentation - Paper for documents - Requirements for permanence".

Transferred to digital printing 2006
ISBN: 90-6203-620-1
©Editions Rodopi B.V., Amsterdam 1984
Printed in the Netherlands

FOREWORD

The Catharina Schrader Stichting was responsible for the idea of producing an English edition of the memoirs of Vrouw Catharina Schrader to coincide with the 21st International Congress of the International Confederation of Midwives held in The Hague in August, 1987. This volume is based largely on the Dutch edition which appeared 1984, *C.G. Schrader's Memoryboeck van de Vrouwens. Het notitieboek van een Friese vroedvrouw 1693-1745.*

The authors would like to acknowledge the contributions of the Catharina Schrader Stichting, who made the publication of this volume and the previous Dutch editions possible. They would also like to offer their thanks to the staff members of the Medisch Encyclopedisch Instituut, Vrije Universiteit, Amsterdam: A.A.G. Ham for her typing work and J.J. van Heel for assistance with proof-reading and the transcription of the manuscript.

Hilary Marland
G.J. Kloosterman
M.J. van Lieburg

TABLE OF CONTENTS

M.J. van Lieburg
CATHARINA SCHRADER (1656-1746) AND HER NOTEBOOK

In all respects the diary of the Frisian midwife Catharina Schrader, first published under the Dutch title "Memoryboeck van de Vrouwens",[1] can be regarded as an exceptional source for the history of obstetrics and the development of midwifery, in particular in The Netherlands. A general introduction to the manuscript, the life and times of its author, and the practice of midwifery may precede here the presentation of Vrouw Schrader's memoirs, the most interesting part of the notebook, to the English-speaking audience.

1. The life of Catharina Geertruida Schrader

Catharina Geertruida (originally in German: Gertraut) Schrader was born at the beginning of September, 1656 in Bentheim, in North-West Germany, the oldest daughter of Friedrich Schrader and Gertrud Nibberich.[2] Vrouw Schrader's father was attached as a tailor to the court of Earl Ernst Wilhelm (1623-1693), who had governed the county of Bentheim since 1643. The county suffered not only from the after effects of the Thirty Years War (1618-1648), but also from the unconventional conduct of the Earl himself.[3]

This political and religious unrest was certainly the main reason behind the move of several members of the family of Friedrich Schrader to Leiden in The Netherlands in the late 1670s. Vrouw Schrader had at least four brothers and a sister. The first brother, Ernst E. Wilhelm (1654-1735), can be traced back to the late 1670s in Leiden, where Catharina also lived till the middle of May, 1682, when she moved back to Bentheim.

On 7 January of the following year Vrouw Schrader married the 29 year old barber-surgeon, Ernst Wilhelm Cramer.[4] There are several indications that this was Ernst Wilhelm's second marriage, and that he had already been in practice in Hallum in Friesland. Initially, the couple stayed in Bentheim, where two daughters were born, Geertrud Elisabeth and Anna Elisabeth. Around 1686 the family moved to Hallum. While living in Hallum the couple had four more children: Jan Frederik, Hendrick, Anna Magdalena and an unnamed daughter. Shortly after the birth of the last child, on 4 February, 1691, Vrouw Schrader's husband died; "my good, learned and highly esteemed, and by God and the people loved husband",[5] and she was left a widow with six young children. Years of hardship followed. In January, 1693, just one year after the death of her husband, Vrouw Schrader set up in practice as a midwife, in addition to her surgical (most likely gynaecological) activities. Her professional work will be discussed in the following chapter.

Almost three years later, in the last week of December, 1695, Vrouw Schrader left the countryside of Hallum for the town of Dokkum, where her children would have the opportunity to attend at the Grammar School. On 26 March, 1713 Vrouw Schrader's daughter married Tjeerd Higt (1690-1761?), an orphan who had been brought up by his uncle, the gold and silversmith, Thomas Higt (1649-1720), who played a leading role in the local government of Dokkum. On 22 February, 1713, one month before the marriage of their children, Thomas Higt took Catharina Geertruida Schrader in marriage.

There followed eight quiet years of marriage for Vrouw Schrader. Her midwifery practice was reduced to only a few deliveries, mostly of family members. Regarding the social position of Thomas Higt, the family were well-placed, which can also be concluded from the financial details given in Schrader's notebook. Both daughters meant a great deal to their aged mother, especially following the death of Thomas Higt in 1720, when she was again left a widow. The second daughter was married to her nephew, Johannes Henricus Schrader, who was called to the ministry in the neighbourhood of Dokkum. In 1718 she assisted with the delivery of her first grandchild. Later Vrouw Schrader followed the career of her grandchildren with close interest and satisfaction. One of them was appointed rector of the Grammar School in Alkmaar and gained national fame as a man of letters, two became ministers in Friesland, another was appointed to a lectureship in history and elocution at the University of Franeker.[6]

Even well into old age, Vrouw Schrader remained in robust health. She makes little reference in the notebook to sickness or the infirmities of old age. In February, 1733 she noted that she was "very ill from a sickness which had affected almost everyone". But even then she was willing to answer a call to assist with a delivery. It is certain that Vrouw Schrader remained active in the practice of midwifery till the end of her life. When on 7 February, 1745 she recorded a delivery for the last time, she was 88 years old. On 30 October, 1746 Catharina Schrader died aged 90 in Dokkum.

2. The manuscript of Vrouw Schrader's notebook and memoirs

The "Memoryboeck van de Vrouwens" covers the period from 9 January, 1693 to 7 February, 1745. Originally the manuscript consisted of nine copy books, described by Vrouw Schrader as "my writing books".

One of these copy books is entitled "Memoryboeck van de Vrouwens" (Notebook of the Women). The relatively stable handwriting can be easily read and gave rise to no serious problems in the transcription; the only problems were connected with punctuation, which Vrouw Schrader used very sparingly. She always used very short sentences, sometimes consisting of only one word, such as "hastig" (make haste) or "lof" (praise). Moreover, Vrouw Schrader wrote in a language which gives clear witness to her German background and a strong Frisian influence.

Vrouw Schrader mostly updated her notebook on the date when she had been called to assist with a delivery. But what motivated Vrouw Schrader to take the trouble to keep her notebook updated in such great detail? Apart from the reasons of financial administration and patient registration, in her memoirs Vrouw Schrader also mentions the possibility of the notebook being used as a guide for her successors in practice of midwifery, including her own daughter. The notebook contains more than details of births, fees and patients. At the end of every year Vrouw Schrader balanced the books, noting down income and expenses and giving the total number of deliveries. She also adopted the habit of opening every new year with a prayer. Besides the notebook, Vrouw Schrader kept a second administration book until 1712, to record her surgical and gynaecological practice.

3. The financial position of Vrouw Schrader

At the end of every case written up in the notebook Vrouw Schrader added the fee requested or received, and in this way kept the books other midwifery practice. At the end of every year she recorded the balance. She was not only paid by the parents of the child, but also, for example, by the grandfather or grandmother (see case 2978).[7] In many cases Vrouw Schrader received no fee at all; in other cases she was paid partly or wholcly in kind; for instance, by a shoemaker, who gave her a pair of slippers and a tradesman, who expressed his appreciation by giving her a pot of shrimps. In the margin the names of patients are sometimes given who had still not paid; in 1709 the list of creditors took up a whole page!

From her notes it appears that Vrouw Schrader obtained her income from various sources. Along with the revenues from her midwifery practice, there were also fees from her gynaecological and surgical practices, profits from the sale of medicines, the interest on bonds and loans, and the proceeds of house letting, etc.[8]

For the years 1720 to 1745 fewer numerical details are given. If we believe her calculations, in the years 1712 to 1733 Vrouw Schrader received 4200 guilders in fees for obstetric assistance and only 1000 guilders for "doctoring and surgery". In any case, it is certain that after the death of her second husband Vrouw Schrader was in a good financial position; Van Kammen found a total of five houses in the name of Vrouw Schrader!

4. The extent and geographical range of Vrouw Schrader's practice

The total number of annual deliveries attended by Vrouw Schrader is given in figure 1 for the period 1693 to 1745. It is possible to distinguish four distinct periods in the life of Vrouw Schrader in this figure: (a) the Hallum period 1693-1695, (b) the years as a widow in Dokkum 1696-1712, (c) the years of her second marriage 1713-1720, and (d) the second period as a widow in Dokkum 1720-1745.

The number of deliveries recorded in the first period totalled forty. Only eight of these occurred in Hallum. (See plate 3 for topographical details.) The most southerly case was in Wijns in 1693 (see case 3), while the tedious journey to Ameland (De Nes) in October, 1694 (case 35) constituted the northern-most limit of her practice. The long journeys and often lengthy sojourn with the patients, obliged Vrouw Schrader to stay away from home regularly for a long period of time, with her six children left behind, the eldest being only ten years old. These factors help explain her departure to Dokkum in the last week of 1695.

In Dokkum Vrouw Schrader was able to build up a large practice in a short period of time, with an average of 120 deliveries per annum in the period 1698 to 1712. Elsewhere, a demographic analysis of these figures will be published at a later date.

Ten per cent of the 1993 deliveries attended in the second period took place outside of Dokkum; most of them were located within a radius of four kilometers around Dokkum. (Vrouw Schrader gives one reason for travelling so long a distance in the memoirs, see case 1975.) In almost all cases, Vrouw Schrader was confronted in the more distant places by more complicated deliveries.

Only twelve deliveries took place in the third period (1712-1720). Vrouw Schrader described this period in her own words, "in my married state sometimes assisted a person in distress". Three of these cases were attendances at the deliveries of her daughters.

The fourth and last period of Vrouw Schrader's practice differs in many respects from the second period. Firstly, the management of the practice was much less uniform than in the years 1696 to 1712. During the first three years she resumed her practice steadily. In the following 22 years she delivered an average of seventy births per year. Secondly, the two periods differed with respect to the proportion of normal and exceptional deliveries. From figure 1 it is clear that by the second period the accent has shifted to "abnormal" cases. The first reason for this shift in emphasis, is

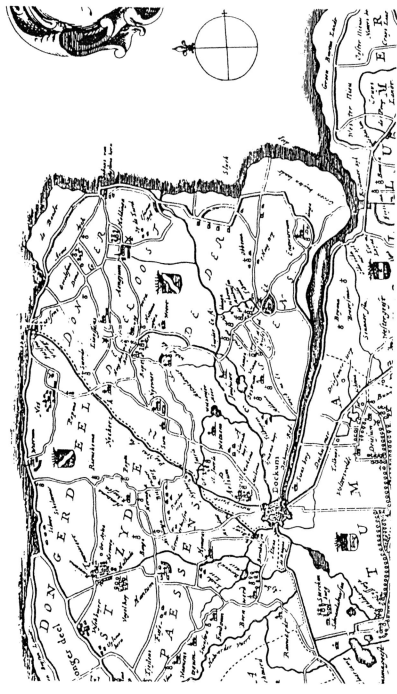

Map of Friesland. From: Chr. Schotanus, *Beschrijvinge van de Heerlyckheydt van Frieslandt tusschen 't Flie end de Lauwers*, 1664.

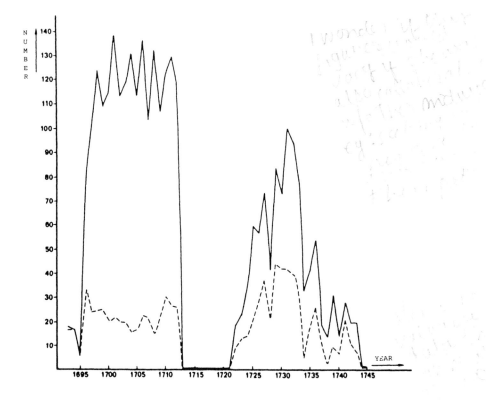

Figure 1. Annual number of deliveries assisted by Vrouw Schrader. A dotted line represents the cases with a more detailed description.

that in the years following 1712 Vrouw Schrader generally made more extensive case notes. It can be suggested that Schrader became more aware of the value of her notes as a rich source of case histories and as a educational tool. The second reason is explained by Kloosterman (hereafter), namely that Vrouw Schrader, because of her special reputation, was called more often to pathological cases.

Thirdly, there was in shift in the balance between Vrouw Schrader's urban and rural practice. Out of the 1027 deliveries taking place in the fourth period, only 6 per cent took place outside Dokkum. Vrouw Schrader's old age would have placed limitations on her ability to travel. A closer examination makes it clear that most of the deliveries she attended outside Dokkum were special in some way. So, for example, out of the 13 journeys to Ternaard, seven were to attend at the births of her grandchildren, and two of the visits to Rinsumageest were paid to her close friend

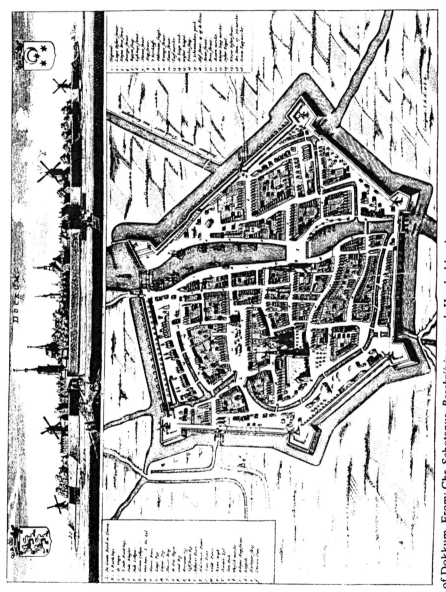

Map of Dokkum. From: Chr. Schotanus, *Beschrijvinge van de Heerlyckheydt van Frieslandt tusschen 't Flie end de Lauwers*, 1664.

Heert, a captain under the Prince of Orange, who she stayed with for three or four weeks, and from whom she received a considerable fee.

Between 1737 and her eightieth anniversary in 1744, one can see that Catharina Schrader purposefully restricted her practice. During these years the average number of deliveries attended amounted to 21 a year. Obviously she was finding it an increasing strain to attend at childbirths. In the middle of 1744 she uttered the lamentation "if this will now be the last for me, The Lord knows. I hope yes". Immediately after this she adds the resigned statement "It will be so". It looks as though Vrouw Schrader finally concluded her practice in 1744, at the beginning of the new year. In 1745 she attended her very last birth, a complicated delivery of the wife of Ype Classen, whom she had managed to deliver of premature twins on an earlier occasion.

5. Dokkum

The town of Dokkum played such an important role in the notebook and memoirs that it warrants a separate section. In the 17th and 18th centuries the old walled town of Dokkum was the communications and trade centre of the north of Friesland,[9] earning this position by reason of its access to the Lauwerszee and because it was situated on important cart tracks and canal paths. On several occasions Vrouw Schrader assisted with the deliveries of women travelling to or from Dokkum, who happened to give birth in the town.

Consequently Dokkum took a central position in the economic life of the region. There was a weekly market, a fish market, particularly for shrimps, and after 1713 a livestock market. Dokkum's role as a sea town is reflected many times in the notebook by the presence of Greenland and East India sailors, skippers and herring fishermen; there was also a shipyard and an old Admiralty House.

Dokkum played a similar role in the religious life of the region, and in teaching and education. Vrouw Schrader's relatives in the ministry have already been mentioned. Out of the non-Protestant religions, only the Baptists or Mennonites, who formed an important religious group, were mentioned in the notebook.[10] Vrouw Schrader was called six times to deliver the wife of Jan Klaasz. de Gorter, "Mennonite preacher and threadwinder" (see, for example, case 1810).

Dokkum society around 1700 is depicted in a special way by the many nicknames given by Vrouw Schrader to her patients and their husbands: Egbert klungel (bungler), Elske kop-af (head off), Mag-lekker-beetjes (nice-little-pieces), Gertie scheefhals (lopsided neck), smerige (dirty) Afke Moy, "Ramsnös" (ram's nose), Klaas kluitjeboer (clod-farmer), Harm rokjager (skirt chaser), Jan potje-pantje (pots and pans), Afke prater (talker), Klaas professor and Anna met de wratten (with the warts) are just a few examples.

6. Vrouw Schrader's clientele

Vrouw Schrader's practice of mentioning the occupation of the husband of her patients and the fees they had to pay enables us to build up a clear picture of the social and economic situation of her clientele. The occupations of the head of the household recorded in the memoirs (see hereafter, table of families) illustrates the diverse background of Vrouw Schrader's clientele, who were drawn from all levels of society.

A categorisation of the fees received by Schrader, shows that generally she fixed a fee for each family she attended. For example, the baker, Sytze Jacobs, paid the amount of three guilders for each of the nine deliveries she assisted with. Schrader received her highest fee of 66 guilders in 1698 from the nobleman, Ernst van Aylva. Other deliveries in the same family yielded around 50 guilders. The same fee was paid by Aylva's son, when Schrader stayed for six weeks at the home of the patient. Vrouw Schrader's remark in her notebook, that during this period "she passed over 10 women", illustrates the relatively large size of the payment.

Fees of between 20 and 50 guilders were received only rarely, when attending the wives of high army functionaries, such as a rittmaster (captain of horse) and an infantry captain. Among the town officials there were some leading citizens who could afford a fee of 4 guilders or more: the town clerks of Dokkum, the bailiff and the mayors. She was usually paid a ducat for deliveries in the homes of legal officers. After a heavy delivery the lawyer, Steenwick, paid twice this amount, which illustrates some relationship between workload and remuneration. Ministers belonged to the same category, all paying something in the region of 7 guilders. The much lower fees received by Vrouw Schrader from members of the medical profession reflects the lower status of this group within the learned professions.[11] In the category of trades some occupations were exceptional in that they permitted the payment of a high fee, such as the gold- and silversmiths and some merchants. Most members of these occupational groups paid three guilders or less.

These figures warrant more detailed examination. In any case a careful interpretation is necessary. For example, patients living outside Dokkum also sometimes had to pay Vrouw Schrader's travelling expenses. Moreover, special circumstances could influence the fixing of the fee. This was obviously the case for the baker, Jan Teircks, in whose household Vrouw Schrader attended 13 deliveries, six of his first wife, and seven "heavy births" of the second (see case 2469).

7. The notebook as a mirror of daily life

In her notebook Vrouw Schrader not only gives administrative details and obstetrical comments about the births she attended, but again and again gives the reader a glimpse into the social background of her patients, cultural life around 1700 and her own emotions concerning her work.

Vrouw Schrader refers not only to the current date of the cases she attended (shifting from the old to the new style in 1701), but also mentioned Catholic holy days and saint days, which is surprising given Vrouw Schrader's denomination. References to Epiphany, Shrove Tuesday, Candlemas, Corpus Christi and All Saints Day reflects, however, the popular culture of the 17th and 18th centuries, where in spite of protest of orthodox Calvinist ministers, the celebration of these days continued. The celebration of saints days can be connected to the annual feast of the guilds, which originated from the commemoration of protective saints. For example, Vrouw Schrader mentions Saint Matthew, protector of bricklayers and carpenters, Saint Jacob, protector of the pilgrims, and Saint Bartholomew, patron of the guild of silversmiths, to which guild Vrouw Schrader's husband and son-in-law belonged.

An example of Schrader's recording of social life is found in case 3 of the memoirs, where Schrader talks about family strife and anxieties concerning the loss of inheritance following the birth of a child. Other cases describe instances of alcohol abuse, unwanted children, and even infanticide, which has been shown to be a widespread phenomenon in the 17th and 18th centuries.[12] In one case we know from legal sources that Vrouw Schrader was involved as an expert witness in a process against a mother who was accused of drowning "the little and innocent child". She explained the progress of the childbed to the lawyers, referring to the lunacy of the mother. Puerperal psychoses were obviously still largely unrecognized. In her memoirs Vrouw Schrader also writes about insanity being caused by tobacco fumes (see case 671).

In addition, the notebook and memoirs bring us into touch with the morality surrounding marriage, and the folklore and superstitions surrounding pregnancy, delivery and childbed of Vrouw Schrader's times. Many unmarried patients are recorded in the notebook, varying in age from "a little girl of 16" to "a sleeped-on-spinster of 40". Promises of marriage proved to play an important role, which allowed pre-marital intercourse to take place, although experience showed that such promises were broken many times. Vrouw Schrader noted down with some precision when a child had been born less than nine months after the marriage. Some children are described as "bastards", some mothers as "whores".

PRAYER OF VROUW SCHRADER (1727)

Here begins again in the name of The Lord the year 1727.

Oh Lord, it is again that I was sent for this purpose by way of Your Godly providence to help my fellow men. So give me then again with this new year new force and strength in my body in my great old age. And so if, Lord, it cannot exist in Your favour and forethought, so send me the means to come out. After all You Lord have decided everything about man, what shall befall him: for better or worse. My eyes are then on You, oh Lord. Help me then again when my fellow men are afflicted with fear and distress. Stay then at my right hand when I take refuge with You. Hear my prayer quickly just like in the days of old. And that I may glorify Your great name. And bless. Not us, oh Lord, but Your name receives all honour, praise, respect and glory to all eternity. Save me from coming across such people, that You wish to make unhappy. Give then if it so pleases You, wisdom, reason, strength. This Your servant beseeches.

Amen, it is so.

Concerning pregnancy, Vrouw Schrader gives much evidence of her strong belief in the role of maternal imagination. In case 2075 of the memoirs she even asks her patient "if something had played on her senses" (see also 1672). She also questioned the behaviour of mothers during pregnancy, which is clearly shown in case 153 of the memoirs. Popular folklore and superstition are intermingled when Schrader talks about "vlygers" and "sugers" (see 525 and 1671).

With respect to the delivery itself, the notebook illustrates the important role of neighbours and friends in the birthing chamber. This was especially true with respect to Dokkum, where the so-called "duty to one's neighbours" was officially enforced.[13] "Come, let us fetch friends and neighbours. I must help you immediately", Schrader ordered to one of her patients in 1698 (see 282). A second example is given in case 1795, where Vrouw Schrader sent all the neighbours home, while in case 661 the mother died "in the presence of all her friends". The active involvement of birth attendants is demonstrated in case 1671. She gives little information on the customs surrounding the lying-in period, only mentioning the consumption of caudle (see 1795).

Vrouw Schrader's innermost feelings and emotions, and her religious experiences, are expressed most clearly in the prayers which she made at the commencement of every year. Her first prayer (1697) already contains, for all its briefness, the three essentials which appeared in all her later prayers: the call for God's "beloved blessing", a prayer for "protection against accidents" and the desire for "the people to receive favour". The choice of her words reveals that Schrader was well-versed in the Scriptures; some prayers are made up of a chain of citations from the Bible. She mentions her patients as "fellow-men" (see the prayer of 1727), the "wretched that I have to see" and those "who are in misery and need". Outwardly Vrouw Schrader showed great courage, but inwardly she had her weaker moments, praying for "deliverance when in my pleading I inwardly pour out my prayer to You". Moreover, as the years passed her bodily condition became an important feature of her prayers. In the last prayer she talks about her great old age, in which God is asked to give her "bodily strength to assist her fellow-men in their need".

8. Vrouw Schrader and the obstetric profession

The notebook of Vrouw Schrader helps us clarify some aspects of the complicated and still little-known structure of the obstetric profession during the 17th and 18th centuries.[14]

First of all, Vrouw Schrader gives some insight into the way she became a midwife by describing her sense of vocation, and her being called by The

Lord to this "weighty affair". The most important obstacles to her responding to this call was the burden of the vocation and the consideration "that is was for me and my friends below my dignity". In her prayers she talks about "this heavy duty", "the work of my vocation" and about the work "Your hand has imposed on me".

Many aspects of her professional role are highlighted in case 16 of the memoirs. Firstly, it shows that already at the beginning of her career Vrouw Schrader felt herself fully competent for the practice of midwifery. She tried to solve all the problems which confronted her "with everything that art required". The question immediately arises as to just how Vrouw Schrader acquired this obstetrical knowledge and these techniques. Taking into account her own cultural and educational background and the surgical profession of her husband, it is likely that she was acquainted to some degree with obstetrical literature. Jacobus Ruffen's *The book of the midwife* (" 't Boeck van de vroet-wijfs", 1591), which was still being re-issued in the 1690s, and *The birth of mankind* ("Der swangern Frauwen und Hebammen", also known in Dutch under the title "Het kleyn vroetwijffs-boeck"), which was re- printed until the middle of the 18th century, can be mentioned in this context. Moreover, the books of Louise Bourgeois and Justine Dittrichs were available in Dutch translations. The well-known books of Francois Mauriceau, Paul Portal and Cornelis Solingen were more oriented towards surgical practice. It is certain that Vrouw Schrader studied the famous book of Hendrik van Deventer, *New Improvements in the Art of Midwifery* ("Manuale Operatien zijnde een Nieuw Ligt voor Vroed-meesters en Vroed-vrouwen", 1701), which is evidenced by the use of the term "lopsided womb" (see Kloosterman). Professional slang or termini technici are seldom used by Vrouw Schrader.

Concerning the use of instruments, the application of enemas, "fomentation" and other skills, Vrouw Schrader must have learned much from the practice of her husband. During the 17th century surgeons's wives were in general directly involved in the practices of their husbands, caring for patients following treatment, assisting in various procedures and keeping the "shop" while their husbands were visiting patients. A well-known example is Hendrik van Deventer's wife, who is said to have had some knowledge of manual techniques and to have assisted in the deliveries of several women.[15]

However, Vrouw Schrader's education and social background differed considerably from that of the typical midwife in the Dutch Republic. The tirades contained in the writings of "enlightened" men-midwives and medical doctors leave us in no doubt about the average midwife, although a certain degree of exaggeration was involved as an unfavourable image helped in the maintenance of the dominant position of male obstetricians.

Also, Vrouw Schrader herself does not speak in a very flattering way about her colleagues. In case 16 she relates how a rival midwife tortured the patient (see also 219, 671, 1975 and 2347). Elsewhere she judged her colleagues as being "a pupil", an incompetent (see 420: "was not able to help her in a proper way"; also case 2116), as "dreadful know-nothings" or as "a messy bungler" (see 2116) and sometimes as being unwilling; on one occasion she describes their results as "spoiled work" (see 2404).

In many cases Vrouw Schrader was called upon after other midwives had failed to complete the delivery. Obviously, she remembered in particular these cases in her memoirs.[16] Sometimes she was fetched on the demand of the woman herself (see 2347). In the case under consideration (number 16) she complied regretfully with the demands of the parturient woman to "fetch another midwife". But finally, she could no longer endure the torturing of the woman, and intervened (see also 74).

Although some rivalry was involved, one should not paint too sombre a picture of the relationship between Vrouw Schrader and her colleagues. The most close relationships were formed with the town midwives. In 1733 her colleague, Feychien Schregardus (who had been assisted at her own deliveries by Vrouw Schrader!) replaced her during her sickness; ten years later the same town midwife was called to assist the aged Vrouw Schrader (who was then 86) to enable her to take a rest.

The second aspect of case 16 concerned the midwives's relations with surgeons and medical doctors. By the end of the 17th century representatives both of the medical and surgical professions were increasingly active in the field of obstetrics. From Schrader's notebook we can build up a picture with the following distinctive features. In obstetric cases the medical doctor could give advice, which was executed by midwives so long as "hand craft" was sufficient. For instrumental help a surgeon had to be called in. Because the separation between medicine and surgery was not so distinctive as has been generally suggested, many medical doctors having followed a surgical training or even being active as surgeons (Solingen and Van Deventer were examples of this), this instrumental help was also provided by medical doctors. In case 16 Vrouw Schrader decided to call "a surgeon ... to avoid all scandal", and asked for Theodorus Winter, a medical doctor and surgeon. Elsewhere she mentions Cornelis Eysma (see 1250), but his role was limited to the prescription of an enema. The status of a certain "Mr." or "Dr." Van den Berg remains unclear (see case 1795). However, Vrouw Schrader's case must have been complicated by the fact that she was obviously acting as a surgeon as well.

In Dokkum Vrouw Schrader co-operated closely with two surgeons: before 1702 with Mr. Pieter Vanij (see 72, 74 and 153) and later with Mr. Frans Berger (see 2047 and 2594). The fact that she acted as midwife to the families of medical doctors and surgeons in Dokkum, amongst whom was the president of the local surgeon's guild, demonstrates that Vrouw Schrader's inter-professional relationships were good. The same holds true for Vrouw Schrader's relationship with the apothecaries of Dokkum, who provided her with medicaments for use in her practice.

Vrouw Schrader's professional situation forms the backdrop for a closer description of her obstetrical activities. In case 16 her functions were confined to an examination of the position of the child. Elsewhere she mentions the internal examination (see case 2313), the rupturing of the membranes, and the making and stimulation of the opening, whether by "hand art" or by fomenting, or both (see 525 and 2596). Vrouw Schrader also used fomentation and poultices for afflictions occurring during childbed and for general complaints (see 643, 1671 and 2192). In one case she combines a poultice with a tincture of myrrh and aloes (see 1831). She must also have had some pharmaceutical knowledge, as shown by the notes recording surgical practices, the cases in which she stimulates the delivery of the child or the afterbirth, stops flooding (see 2979) or relieves pain.

Repeatedly Vrouw Schrader came into contact with pastoral care (see case 72). In 1740 she was called to a patient whom the minister had already prayed for (see 2979); one day later she met the local minister in the delivery room (see 2980).

The normal injunction on the use of instruments by midwives did not apply to Vrouw Schrader. The statement that she had taken her instruments with her because she expected difficulties (see 1485) makes it clear that Vrouw Schrader had her own collection of instruments. In any case, her bag contained a "razor" (see 1157 and 1626), an enema syringe (see 1030 and 1810), a catheter (see 1810), bandages (see 606 and 1880) and obstetrical hooks. The use of these instruments is illustrated in several cases.[17] While she makes frequent mention of the delivery bed, Vrouw Schrader never refers to the use of the delivery stool.

The end of case 16 focuses on an as yet unmentioned aspect of Vrouw Schrader's personality: her professional pride and awareness of her own abilities. The "solemn testimonial and great honour" awarded to her by the doctor in attendance evidently gave her a feeling of pride. But what bearing should a sentence such as that occurring in case 581, where she noted down "Had it immediately to [the] great astonishment of all those who were present", have on our interpretation of Vrouw Schrader's personality?

9. Epilogue

The notebook of Vrouw Schrader still calls forth feelings of amazement and admiration. Certainly Vrouw Schrader's notes offer a necessary counter-weight to all those historical studies in which 17th- and 18th-century obstetrics, especially the position of midwives, is depicted in somber tones. The scope of this volume has been limited to the presentation of Vrouw Schrader's notebook to the English audience. This edition will preface further research into the history of midwifery in the Dutch Republic.

NOTES

1. M.J. van Lieburg (ed.), *C.G. Schrader's Memoryboek van de Vrouwens. Het notitieboek van een Friese vroedvrouw 1693-1745. Met een verloskundig commentaar van Prof.dr. G.J. Kloosterman*, Amsterdam: Editions Rodopi, 1984 (1st and 2nd editions) and 1985 (3rd edition).
2. For detailed information about the sources, see M.J. van Lieburg, "Het Memoryboeck als medisch-historische bron", in: Van Lieburg, *C.G. Schrader's Memoryboeck* (note 1), 1-46.
3. See W.F. Visch, *Geschiedenis van het Graafschap Bentheim*, Zwolle: J.L. Zeehuisen, 1820 and J.C. Möller, *Geschichte der vormaligen Grafschaft Bentheim von den älteren Zeiten bis auf unsere Tage*, Lingen 1879.
4. See for the family Kramer (Cramer): *Bijblad Nederlandse Leeuw* 2 (1954) 153-174.
5. See the beginning of her memoirs.
6. See for J. Schrader: A.J. van der Aa, *Biografisch Woordenboek*, (Haarlem 1853) vol. 6, col. 149 and P.C. Molhuysen, *Nieuw Nederlands Biografisch Woordenboek* (Leiden: A.W. Sijthoff, 1937), vol. 10, col. 894-895.
7. Numbers are only mentioned when they are recorded in the memoirs. All case-numbers correspond with the numbers in the Dutch-edition.
8. See Table 1 in the Dutch edition (note 1).
9. See W.K. v.d. Veen, "Dokkum en de omliggende dorpen", *It Beaken* 16 (1954) 220-223.
10. S. Blaupot ten Cate, *Geschiedenis der Doopsgezinden in Friesland*, Leeuwarden: W. Eekhoff, 1839.
11. Cf. W.Th. Frijhoff, "Non satis dignitatis. Over de maatschappelijke status van geneeskundigen tijdens de Republiek", *Tijdschr. Geschiedenis* 96 (1983) 379-406.
12. L. van Nierop, "De keuren tegen het ombrengen van jong-gebore kinderen in de 17e en 18e eeuw", *Maandblad Amstelodamum* 46 (1959) 154-155 and H. Rodega, *Kindestötung und Verheimlichung der Schwangerschaft. Ein sozialgeschichtliche und medizinsoziologische Untersuchung mit Einzelfallanalysen*, Herzogenrath: Murken-Altrogge, 1981.
13. See S.J. van der Molen, "Men zal de naasten bereid vinden (burenplicht in Friesland in de 18e en 19e eeuw)", *De Vrije Fries* 46 (1964) 28-61.
14. Cf. E.H. Ackerknecht, "Zur Geschichte der Hebammen", *Gesnerus* 31 (1974) 181-192; J. Gélis, "Sages-femmes et accoucheurs: l'obstétrique populaire aux XVIIe et XVIIIe siècle", *Annales Econ. Sociétés Civilisations* 32 (1977) 927-957 and

22

the same, "Regard sur l'Europe médicale des Lumières: la collaboration inter-
nationale des accoucheurs et la formation des sages-femmes au XVIIIe siècle",
Abhand. Gesch. Med. Naturwiss. 39 (1980) 279-299. For England see the literature,
given by Hilary Marland.

15. See H.J. Lamers, *Hendrik van Deventer Medicinae Doctor, 1651-1724. Leven en
Werken*, Assen: Van Gorcum, 1946.
16. See the cases 18, 20, 161, 219, 420, 606, 671, 743, 971, 1296, 1485, 1728, 1743, 1831,
1847, 1888, 1943, 1975, 1984, 2047, 2119, 2137, 2347, 2404 and 2980.
17. See numbers 74, 153, 872, 968, 1485 and 2183.

TABLE OF FAMILIES, RECORDED IN THE MEMOIRS
Compiled by F.A. van Lieburg

A = Case from the memoirs
B = Corresponding number in the Dutch edition
C = Place of the birth
D = Date of birth
E = Date of marriage
F = Date of baptism
G = Profession of husband
H = Fee
(*) = Twin / (**) = Triplet

Case-numbers 365 and 486, 2571 and 2822, and 2809 and 2933 belong to one family.

A	B	C	D	E	F	G	H
1	1	Hallum	9-1-1693	4-5-1690	15-1-1693	unknown	2-2
2	3	Wijns	26-2-1693	unknown	unknown	unknown	2-14
3	16	Marrum	2-11-1693	unknown	none	merchant	3-3
4	18	De Leie	31-12-1693	unknown	unknown	horseman	unknown
5	20	Dokkum	27-1-1694	unknown	unknown	unknown	1-2
6	35	Nes (Ameland)	6-10-1694	source lost	unknown	skipper	5-0
7	39	Dokkum	16-12-1695	unknown	unknown	unknown	?
8	54	Dokkum	12-3-1696	unknown	unknown	skipper	2-10
9	72	Dokkum	22-6-1696	unknown	unknown	wagon maker	3-0
10	74	Dokkum	13-7-1696	unknown	none	carpenter	6-6
11*	88	Dokkum	17-8-1696	unknown	23-8-1696	cord maker	2-15
12	89	Dokkum	18-8-1696	unknown	23-8-1696	tile maker	2-4
13*	150	Dokkum	6-5-1697	unknown	9-5-1697	miller	1-10
14	153	Dokkum	17-5-1697	unknown	unknown	innkeeper	3-3
15**	161	Oostrum	30-6-1697	source lost	source lost	farmer	1-2
16	219	Dokkum	28-12-1696	unknown	unknown	farmer	3-0
17*	282	Dokkum	3-7-1698	unknown	unknown	baker	2-2
18	365	Dokkum	15-2-1699	unknown	none	painter	3-3
19	418	Dokkum	16-9-1699	12-3-1699	none	soldier	1-13
20	420	Dokkum	24-9-1699	unknown	unknown	linen worker	1-10
21	423	Dokkum	4-10-1699	unknown	unknown	town crier	5-0
22	485	Dokkum	12-3-1700	5-3-1699	13-2-1700	shoemaker	1-10
23	486	Dokkum	13-3-1700	unknown	unknown	painter/thread winder	33

24	521	Rinsumageest	18-7-1700	unknown	unknown	labourer	1-8
25	525	Dokkum	30-7-1700	unknown	unknown	skipper	3-0
26	581	Akkerwoude	27-1-1701	source lost	source lost	unknown	2-0
27	595	Dantuma-woude	1-3-1701	source lost	none	unknown	2-0
28	597	Dokkum	4-3-1701	unknown	unknown	wool-comber	1-10
29	606	Dokkum	23-3-1701	4-11-1697	none	baker	22
30	643	Dokkum	2-7-1701	unknown	none	smith	4-0
31	661	Dokkum	1701	unknown	unknown	merchant	2-10
32	671	Driesum	2-10-1701	source lost	none	weaver	18
33	743	Rinsuma-geest	4-5-1702	none	21-5-1702	none	4-0
34*	796	Dokkum	12-10-1702	unknown	11-10-1702	knitter	0-0
35	825	Dantuma-woude	24-1-1703	source lost	21-1-1703	minister	60
36	852	Hantum	..-3-1703	unknown	none	tailor	3-3
37	872	Dokkum	3-6-1703	unknown	unknown	wagon maker	9-3
38	968	Dokkum	10-3-1704	15-4-1703	none	unknown	66
39*	969	Driesum	13-3-1704	source lost	24-3-1704	unknown	2-12
40	971	Joure	13-3-1704	unknown	unknown	unknown	0-0
41*	1024	Dokkum	12-9-1704	8-10-1702	3-8-1704	butcher	3-0
42*	1030	Dokkum	20-9-1704	6-6-1703	unknown	town-beadle	1-18
43	1062	Dokkum	1-12-1704	7-5-1699	none	cord maker	2-0
44	1157	Dokkum	25-10-1705	23-4-1697	unknown	corporal	1-8
45	1211	Oosterwolde	19-3-1706	unknown	source lost	unknown	2-15
46	1233	Driesum	12-6-1706	source lost	unknown	skipper	2-8
47	1250	Dokkum	1-8-1706	unknown	unknown	bricklayer	2-4
48	1296	Hantum	21-12-1706	unknown	none	unknown	1-8
49	1374	Dokkum	3-9-1707	unknown	unknown	potter	1-10
50	1382	Dokkum	15-9-1707	14-1-1703	none	gardener	3-2
51	1485	Werdeburen	19-7-1708	unknown	unknown	labourer	9-9
52	1533	Oostrum	15-11-1708	source lost	none	labourer	1-0
53	1609	Dokkum	9-6-1709	none	unknown	none	2-8
54*	1626	Dokkum	1-8-1709	20-5-1708	none	cooper	2-0
55	1656	Driesum	23-11-1709	source lost	none	carpenter	3-3
56	1671	Dokkum	25-1-1710	unknown	none	copper repairer	5-10
57	1672	Dokkum	5-2-1710	unknown	unknown	corn merchant	2-10
58	1728	Ternaard	6-9-1710	27-10-1709	14-9-1710	verger	2-0
59*	1734	Dokkum	27-9-1710	unknown	19-10-1710	brewer	6-6
60	1743	Hantum	18-10-1710	unknown	unknown	unknown	6-0
61	1795	Nijkerk	10-2-1711	unknown	unknown	unknown	4-10
62	1810	Dokkum	20-3-1711	29-12-1709	none	thread-winder/ preacher	42-0
63	1824	Dokkum	28-4-1711	20-9-1705	19-4-1711	boat builder	3-0
64	1831	Dokkum	11-6-1711	unknown	unknown	labourer	3-0
65	1847	Driesum	3-8-1711	source lost	none	tailor	1-3
66	1880	Ternaard	14-10-1711	[28-4-]1709	none	carrot buyer	5-0
67	1888	Oosterwolde	1-11-1711	unknown	none	unknown	1-2
68	1943	Driesum	11-3-1712	source lost	none	cattle dealer	6-10

69	1975	Dokkum	4-8-1712	unknown	unknown	labourer	2-10
70	1984	Akkerwoude	24-8-1712	unknown	none	unknown	6-0
71	1993	Driesum	7-9-1712	source lost	none	farmer	3-0
72	2047	Dokkum	3-2-1722	unknown	unknown	skipper	0-0
73	2075	Dokkum	21-5-1723	3-5-1722	none	currier	2-0
74*	2090	Dokkum	27-1-1724	28-1-1720	30-1-1724	confectioner	3-3
75	2114	Dokkum	20-9-1724	unknown	unknown	butcher	3-3
76	2116	Dokkum	13-11-1724	3-11-1715	none	girdle maker	unknown
77	2119	Dokkum	8-12-1724	unknown	unknown	merchant	5-0
78	2132	Dokkum	1-3-1725	14-6-1722	none	miller	4-3
79	2137	Dokkum	2-4-1725	28-6-1716	8-4-1725	tailor	2-10
80	2183	Rinsumageest	4-1-1726	source lost	none	dairyman	5-0
81	2185	Ternaard	14-3-1726	16-6-1720	17-3-1726	minister	0-0
82	2192	Dokkum	20-4-1726	6-8-1725	none	town councillor	4-0
83*	2205	Dokkum	3-8-1726	unknown	unknown	smith	3-11
84	2240	Dokkum	3-1-1727	18-11-1725	unknown	potter	3-2
85	2261	Dokkum	13-4-1727	18-6-1724	13-4-1727	dairyman	2-10
86	2265	Dokkum	3-5-1727	unknown	none	mayor	6-11
87**	2292	Dokkum	8-9-1727	17-1-1723	20-9-1727	skipper	4-11
88	2313	Dokkum	14-1-1728	19-2-1722	16-2-1728	turf cutter	2-5
89	2347	Dokkum	23-11-1728	unknown	unknown	baker	3-3
90	2404	Dokkum	26-8-1729	25-7-1728	none	toll keeper	1-10
91	2421	Dokkum	26-11-1729	27-12-1722	none	geneva distiller	44
92	2431	Dokkum	18-12-1729	21-11-1723	unknown	shoemaker	5-0
93	2441	Dokkum	10-2-1730	1-1-1729	12-2-1730	peddler	3-3
94	2465	Dokkum	30-5-1730	3-3-1726	31-5-1730	cooper	3-2
95	2469	Dokkum	11-6-1730	5-7-1722	none	baker	4-10
96	2520	Dokkum	27-2-1731	28-11-1723	28-2-1731	shoemaker	2-0
97	2569	Dokkum	1-8-1731	circa 1710	unknown	geneva distiller	42-15
98	2571	Dokkum	8-8-1731	7-6-1728	12-8-1731	butcher	2-0
99	2594	Dokkum	13-10-1731	unknown	unknown	bargeman	6-0
100	2596	Dokkum	18-10-1731	28-1-1731	28-10-1731	seaman	1-10
101	2598	Hantum	22-10-1731	1-7-1725	unknown	minister	7-0
102*	2626	Dokkum	6-3-1732	22-4-1731	9-3-1732	innkeeper	4-4
103	2640	Dokkum	12-4-1732	26-3-1730	14-4-1732	ship's carpenter	3-10
104	2653	Dokkum	26-5-1732	unknown	2-6-1732	ship's carpenter	3-2
105	2668	Dokkum	28-7-1732	19-9-1723	6-8-1732	labourer	1-2
106	2686	Dokkum	16-9-1732	5-6-1729	none	shoemaker	1-10
107	2771	Dokkum	10-11-1733	unknown	unknown	servant	0-0
108	2809	Dokkum	21-4-1734	19-3-1732	28-4-1734	butcher	3-0
109	2817	Dokkum	1734	22-6-1732	4-8-1734	merchant/skipper	unknown
110	2818	Dokkum	8-8-1734	unknown	22-8-1734	tile labourer	unknown
111	2819	Dokkum	9-8-1734	3-5-1733	15-8-1734	miller	unknown

112	2820	Dokkum	1734	unknown	unknown	shoemaker/	
						tradesman	unknown
113	2821	Dokkum	6-9-1734	25-6-1724	unknown	sailor	unknown
114	2822	Dokkum	20-11-1734	7-6-1728	unknown	butcher	unknown
115	2823	Dokkum	3-2-1735	23-9-1731	6-2-1735	basket maker	unknown
116	2906	Dokkum	28-10-1736	unknown	unknown	tile labourer	1-10
117	2933	Dokkum	21-4-1738	9-3-1732	unknown	butcher	2-10
118	2956	Dokkum	22-5-1739	7-9-1738	24-5-1739	merchant	3-6
119	2969	Dokkum	29-9-1739	14-9-1738	29-9-1739	geneva	
						distiller	30
120	2978	Betterwird	29-2-1740	unknown	unknown	farmer	6-2
121	2979	Aalsum	23-5-1740	30-1-1718	none	schoolmaster	4-0
122	2980	Oostrum	24-5-1740	source lost	none	unknown	9-0

549

1743 den ~~4~~ november op donderday by
Johannes Jellies synde een wagenar en koo
melker syn vrouw eele een jonge dochtij-ie

1743 den 17 desember Sys schutemackers
syn wyf eele schuring en haar verlost
van een dood vervol kint had sy neg
in haar dragt leven gevoelt en moet so
matter tit sucklick gewest, en de moeder
een gesonde vraw het left vrurtian — 2 —

1744 den 19 mart gehult by fryt
pryek macker en Mller syn wyf deers
tans een jong soon —————— 1 —

1745 den 7 febrwary by ~~tpe~~ backr
syn vrouw gehult weror dat het water
de nug wag ist dat ici greelich tag
de mette on hog in de syde sonde het riet
het erfy ver en muft so deirgeboren
en de mei grote verse endies verspart
het en dakter ende de moeder en het
kint venenwilde heer sy gedankt ~~....~~

Page from the Notebook of Vrouw Schrader (folio 549)

G.J. Kloosterman
SOME OBSTETRIC REMARKS ON VROUW SCHRADER'S NOTE-
BOOK AND MEMOIRS

Catharina Schrader lived in a period in which the "trade" or profession
of what we now call obstetrics and gynaecology, a trade which from time
immemorial was considered as the exclusive domain of women, came more
and more into the hands of man-midwives. The idea that women had an
innate and natural talent which enabled them to assist other women during
childbirth was challenged, and midwives increasingly became targets for
accusations in every delivery which had a bad outcome; on the one hand
accused of procrastination, on the other of impatience and aggressive
behaviour, and almost always of ignorance.

Together with Louise Bourgeois (1564-1640) in France, and Justina
Siegemund (1650-1705) in Germany and Jane Sharp (circa 1620-1680) in
England, we can name Catharina Schrader as an example of experienced
midwives who not only excelled by way of their skill and great personal
experience, but who also tried to incorporate into their practice the
discoveries made in an exclusively male world of medicine. All these
midwives wrote books to teach and assist other midwives. Bourgeois wrote
Observations diverses,[1] and this book, published in Paris in 1626, was
translated into Dutch and German. Louise Bourgeois was married to the
surgeon Martin Bourcier (a pupil of the famous Ambroise Paré. She
became the midwife of the French queen Maria de Médicis and assisted the
queen in six deliveries. She wrote e.g. on transverse positions, placenta
praevia and face presentations. She recommended expectant behaviour in
face presentations stating that many of them could been born spontaneously; advise that for almost two centuries was not followed till
Johannes Boër (1789-1835) brought this attitude under general consideration. Siegemund wrote a book in 1686 that was already by 1691 translated
into Dutch by the doctor medicinae et obstetriciae, Cornelis Solingen.[2]
Jane Sharp published *The Midwives Book* in 1671.[3]

There is nevertheless a great difference between the notebook of
Schrader and the books of her colleagues, a difference which makes this
notebook unique in the history of obstetrics. Whereas all of the books gave
descriptions of obstetric cases which were linked to warnings or lessons for
the reader, Schrader gives chronological descriptions of *all* her deliveries.

This enables us to study the frequency of complicated cases and disasters, and also to some extent the outcome of the birth process for mother and child, in the practice of an experienced midwife during a period of 52 years around the turn of the 18th century.

1. Maternal mortality

The modern definition of maternal mortality includes all maternal deaths caused by or connected to pregnancy, and occurring during pregnancy, childbirth and a period of 42 (or 90) days after delivery. As prenatal care did not exist before the end of the 19th century, the first contact with the midwife usually taking place during delivery, the follow-up during the lying-in period also being rather short, we cannot expect Vrouw Schrader's data to be sufficient to produce a figure of maternal mortality comparable with modern criteria. Only figures for deaths occurring during or shortly after the delivery can be given, but even this presents an important and rather unique possibility.

In her memoirs Vrouw Schrader describes 122 "bad and heavy complicated births" to use her own words. We could expect that all cases ending in the death of the mother were mentioned in these memoirs, for nowadays we call these the greatest disaster in obstetrics. And indeed eleven fatal cases are mentioned.

Many readers, taking the line that Vrouw Schrader mentioned all maternal deaths in her memoirs concluded that she had lost only eleven mothers in more than 3000, perhaps even 4000 deliveries and came to a figure for maternal mortality of 3 to $4^o/_{oo}$. This is misleading however. In the notebook we can find nine other cases with a fatal outcome, bringing the maternal mortality rate to 5 to $7^o/_{oo}$.[4]

On the other hand we must keep in mind the fact, that Vrouw Schrader often was regarded as a last resort and asked to help in already lost cases. It is undoubtedly no coincidence that almost all these cases are mentioned in the memoirs (see 16, 35, 671, 1975 and 2980). In the notebook we find only one other case (number 101) in which the mother died before Vrouw Schrader entered the house. Two living children were born in the presence of another midwife. The woman died shortly after the birth of the second child (by haemorrhage?).

This means that Vrouw Schrader was six times asked to help in already lost cases; situations in which the responsibility for the delivery did not rest on her shoulders. If we leave out these cases, and only include maternal deaths in the practice of Vrouw Schrader herself, than the (direct) maternal deaths are 14 in 3017 deliveries, that is $4.6^o/_{oo}$, a figure far better than the suppositions of many authors, writing on obstetrical results in the 17th and 18th centuries; especially, if we keep in mind that the practice of Schrader contained much more pathology than can be expected in a random sample of the population.

Another important fact we like to stress is, that Schrader in her memoirs did not include all cases of maternal mortality. In many situations she regarded a fatal outcome as something that could not have been avoided. If there was nothing to blame in the conduct of the midwife (or the patient and her surrounding) than death was taken as something that had to be accepted as the will of God.

An analysis of the 20 cases of maternal mortality shows, that infection (sepsis puerperalis) has been the most probable explanation in nine cases (see 16, 153, 643, 1671, 2594 and 2822 in the memoirs; and 2187, 2201 and 3052 in the notebook). Case 2822 is almost certainly an example of diffuse intravascular clotting (D.I.C.) caused by a massive introduction of toxins of Gram-negative bacteria into the maternal circulation during the birth of the (living) child. In the other eight cases death came after three days in three cases, after seven and nine days (two cases), twelve days and 21 days. In the first three cases, where death occurred already after three days, we also have to think of (incomplete) rupture of the uterus, since not only the delivery lasted very long (three days) but in all cases the dead child was born artificially by a difficult version and extraction (see 643) or (after perforation of the skull) by means of the crotchet (see 153 and 2594).

In four cases death occurred after seven to 21 days. Prolonged labour with early rupture of the membranes and a difficult artificial delivery is mentioned in one case (notebook 3052); prolonged and difficult labour, together with a subtotal prolapse of the uterus, already in the second half of pregnancy, in case 1671; in case 2201 of the notebook, a difficult manual removal of the placenta was necessary after a prolonged labour and heavy blood loss. In case 16 the day of death is not mentioned, but also in that case there was a very long and difficult labour (in spite of a normal presentation) followed by extraction of the (dead) child with an instrument. In fact there is only one case in more than 3000 deliveries (see 2187 in the notebook) where death of the mother occurred (after seven days) in all probability by sepsis puerperalis after a quick spontaneous labour with a live born child.

In five cases death has to be attributed to a severe haemorrhage. In case 35 by partial retentio placentae after birth of twins; the same thing, also after birth of two (living) children happened in case 101 (notebook). In cases 661 and 2979 there was a placenta praevia totalis. Loss of blood, together with shock by exhaustion, pain and neglect, will have played a part in case 1975.

Case 671 seems to have been a case of eclampsia followed by a cerebral haemorrhage. The day after the birth of the second child of twins there was a strong emotional stimulus and thereafter insults, followed by coma. Died that same day. Some readers have spoken of psychosis puerperalis, but this gives no explanation for the death of the woman. Case 1988, not mentioned in the memoirs, is perhaps not even a maternal death. The woman died, but she was not in labour and died three days after Vrouw Schrader left her, because she was not in labour. The woman complained of very heavy and constant abdominal pain. Perhaps she was not pregnant at all. If she was, than we can think of an abdominal pregnancy or of rupture of an aneurysm. In case 2394 (not in the memoirs) the woman died on the fourth day, after a spontaneous and very quick delivery of a tiny and prematurely born boy. She had a gangrenous leg. Death by infection or massive embolism seems the most probable explanation. In case 2738 (not in the memoirs), after a quick and easy birth mother and child died on the third day. Cause of death stays enigmatic.

In case 2872 (notebook only), after difficult labour, a macerated child was born in breech position. Difficulties with the after coming head. In her notebook she mentions: this died. As she already told that the child was macerated, it is almost certain the mother died. Where and how stays obscure. And in case 2992 (only in the notebook), there was a heavy haemorrhage in pregnancy. Two days later a dead child was born. Was already dead for three days. Premature (seven months). Mother became very ill the day after the spontaneous delivery and died on the tenth day in coma. Heavy headache. Cause uncertain. We could think of sinus thrombosis, the more so, since this was the fourth stillborn child in succession of this woman. A vascular disease with enhanced tendency to thrombosis seems probable. A partial abruptio placentae could explain the haemorrhage.

Summarizing we can say, that in at least nine cases infection has been the most important cause (including one case of D.I.C.). In three of these cases a combination of infection with damage done to the uterus (incomplete rupture?) seems probable. Second comes death by heavy blood loss. Twice during the third stage of labour after birth of twins, twice as a complication of placenta praevia totalis.

There was one case of eclampsia, and two cases of pre-existent vascular disease, ending with thrombosis and/or embolism (see 2394 and 2992, both only in the notebook). In three cases (see 1988, 2738 and 2872, all not in the memoirs) the cause of maternal death stays an enigma. In case 1988 it is not even certain there existed a pregnancy. If so, than we can think of an abdominal pregnancy or the rupture of an abdominal aneurysm. The other two cases give insufficient details for a diagnosis.

The notorious trias for maternal death clearly comes forward. Infection, in combination with artificial deliveries is number one. Then comes haemorrhage. Third: toxaemia with one case of eclampsia and at least two cases of pre-existent vascular disease.

2. Abnormal presentations

In her very first case Catharina Schrader was confronted with an abnormal presentation; she mentions in her notebook that the child came "with his face upwards". It has been wrongly concluded by some commentators that this was a face presentation. A true face presentation was described in case 2137; as proof of this, the child's face was described as being "swollen and puffy". Case 423, where the child came repeatedly with his eyes before the birth canal, was also apparently a face presentation. Four other cases of face presentations were found in the notebook, which were not mentioned in the memoirs. In these cases, Vrouw Schrader describes how the child "came with its face in the birth canal" and "came with its eyes in the birth canal". After the delivery, it is mentioned that the child's "upper lip was terribly swollen" (see 1993, and also 1732, 2131 and 2373, not in the memoirs).

Deliveries where the child "came with its face upwards" were much more frequent. Such cases were recorded at least 16 times in the notebook. In one case Catharina Schrader performed version and extraction (see 2465) and the child survived; in another (see 2185) she was forced to resort to the crotchet, following the death of the child. In all other 14 cases of persistent occiput posterior position ("came with his face upwards") the birth was spontaneous and the children were alive when delivered. In a few cases, however, Schrader wrote of a "difficult", or even "terribly difficult" delivery.

Breech deliveries, nowadays divided into frank breeches and complete or full breeches, not to mention other possible sub-divisions, were not mentioned by Vrouw Schrader by these modern names, but it is not difficult to diagnose the frank breech by the descriptions she gave. If, for example, she writes: came with the buttocks first, the bottom presented in the birth canal, its private parts presented in the birth canal, came doubled up with the feet to the shoulders,then we have to deal with a frank breech.

In the notebook more than 40 cases were found of complete breech and 27 cases of frank breech. Nowadays the number of frank breeches is usually equal to or greater than the number of complete breeches, but it is easy to understand that at the times of Schrader this was very different. This can be explained by the greater number of multiparae; another explanation is that Schrader often was called in for pathological cases, and frank breeches occur more often together with physiological conditions than complete breeches.

It is harder to explain why the total number of breech deliveries (about 2.5 per cent) is lower than we find nowadays. Two explanations can be given: firstly, in many cases of a spontaneous delivery she does not mention the presentation of the child. As many cases of breech delivery are born as smoothly as head presentations and Vrouw Schrader did not consider every case of breech presentation as an indication to interfere, there have been in all probability more cases of breech presentation than are mentioned in her notebook.

In the second place, Vrouw Schrader does not always make a sharp distinction between breech and transverse presentation. If she mentions (see 485): "it lay with his back before the birth canal, then turned it, but had to be born doubled up with his buttocks first", we can think of a transverse position, born ultimately as a frank breech. But it is also possible, that from the beginning this must be considered to have been a frank breech. Other examples in the notebook are cases 2049, 2210 and 2858.

The total number of transverse positions (more than 50) is considerably higher than we find nowadays (more than 2% against less than 0.5%). This is not surprising, given the high number of grand multiparae and the concentration of pathology in her practice.

In 16 cases she mentions prolapse of the cord in her notebook. This rather low number (about 0.5%), can be explained by the fact that mentioning this occurrence is mostly done if this was related to the death of the child, that is in combination with a head or breech presentation. It is probable that in many cases of transverse presentation prolapse of the cord has not been mentioned at all.

3. Placenta praevia

In the same way as Louise Bourgeois and Justina Siegemundin, Vrouw Schrader discovered this complication, now called placenta praevia, by herself. All three midwives came to the conclusion that the best way to handle these extremely dangerous situations consists of delivering the woman as soon as possible. Justina Siegemundin attained this goal by piercing the placenta with a needle to drain away the amniotic fluid. Schrader, in the same way as Louise Bourgeois came by personal experience to the conclusion that she had to remove the placenta first, performing a version and extraction immediately thereafter.

In case 661 Vrouw Schrader lost her patient and came to the conclusion that she had to act quicker, if such a case came in her way another time. In case 1250 she had the opportunity to execute this plan and delivered the woman just in time (to the amazement of Doctor Eysma, who could not believe that a woman could be delivered without labour pains). Several other examples of placenta praevia have been described in the notebook;[5]

in the memoirs she describes only the cases 661, 1250, 2132, 2979 and 2980. The description of case 2980 leaves it uncertain whether this is a case of placenta praevia, but in the notebook is mentioned: "The afterbirth was in front of the child in the mouth of the womb and stuck very fast. Could not remove it completely".

If we consider that only severe cases (total and lateral) of placenta praevia are mentioned, then a frequency of more than $3^o/_{oo}$ is high. Of course we can expect a rather high number of placenta praevia in a practice with more multiparae and more women of rather high age than nowadays. Nevertheless, a certain concentration of pathology in the practice of Vrouw Schrader is certain whereas a mortality rate of 2 in 10 is low for a complication that can be considered as one of the most dangerous complications of pregnancy. The two fatal cases are both mentioned in the memoirs (see 661 and 2980).

4. Perinatal mortality

The modern definition of perinatal mortality includes all fetuses and infants delivered weighing at least 500 gram, or, when birth weight is unavailable, the corresponding gestational age (22 weeks) or body length (25 cm crown-heel). For international comparisons standard perinatal mortality is recommended, in which only fetuses and infants weighing 1000 gram or more (28 weeks, 35 cm crown-heel) are included. Neonatal death includes live born infants dying in the first 168 hours.

It goes without saying that we can not use these definitions in an obstetrical practice of almost three centuries ago. The custom to weigh children started at a much later date than many people realize. Mauriceau, in the fourth edition of his *Traité des Maladies des Femmes grosses* (1694) devotes only a few words on the weight of a newborn and gives as a normal weight 13 to 14 pounds (6500 to 7000 grams).[6] Even if we accept that a medical pound in his times has been 369 gram, even then we come to an absurd outcome. In 1747 Theophilus Lobb (1678-1763),[7] who was writing "A Compendium of the Practice of Physick" asked the man-midwife Phillipson to give him some data on normal birth weight. He got the information that a newborn child weighed 16 pounds and seven ounces (7424 gram), the placenta together with the navel string one pound and four ounces (578 gram). This normal figure for the placenta and umbilical cord proves that the weight for the child is measured to high. Probably the child was weighed after it was swaddled. The first realistic weights of newborns come from the German obstetrician Roederer (1726-1763) in Göttingen who found an average of 3066 grams for the birth weight of boys and 2871 grams for girls. It was only in the second half of the 19th century that weighing newborn babies came into general use.

The same neglect of exact data for weight is also found for data on the duration of pregnancy. It is impossible to make a subdivision in abortion, pre-term, term and post-term labour. The only indications on duration of pregnancy we can find in the memoirs and in the notebook are:

1) abortion; small fruit of three months; miscarriage of twelve weeks. In all 25 cases are mentioned in the notebook and none of them in the memoirs. A figure of less than one percent abortion is far too low. We can assume this figure to have been at least 8 to 10%. This proves that in a great majority no help of a midwife was asked in cases of abortion. That Vrouw Schrader herself did not think much of these early miscarriages appears from the fact that she did not mention any of the 25 cases in her memoirs.

2) In 27 cases she mentions a "fruit of 4, 5 or 6 months" but, once again, none of these cases are considered significant enough to be included in the memoirs. All cases ended well for the mother, all fetuses were stillborn or died shortly after birth. A percentage of almost one percent of these occurrences, not far from the percentage that is found in modern times shows, that these cases, in contradistinction to early abortions, were considered worth while to ask for obstetric assistance.

3) A delivery after a duration of pregnancy of seven-months is mentioned 35 times. Among them were three twins which brings the total number of seven-months children to 38. This is in striking contrast with the fact that only four times a birth of eight-months is mentioned (one twin, thus five children).

From the 38 seven-months children, 24 died (63%), 14 stayed alive. From the five eight-months children, three died, two stayed alive. It is clear that the frequency of eight-months children is much too low. The old adagium of Hippocrates that eight-months children are worse off than seven-months children can have influenced her judgment and that children "that did well" and survived have been considered as mature children.

That duration of pregnancy was not accurately measured and many cases of premature birth were accepted as mature, is also shown by the fact that in 70 twins and two triple pregnancies (see 161 and 2292) she mentions only four times that the pregnancy ended prematurely. This is another proof that the estimation of the duration of pregnancy has been very inaccurate.

From all this it is apparent we cannot use modern subdivisions for prenatal mortality, but an overall figure is possible. In the notebook we find 140 cases of fetal and neonatal death without data on the duration of pregnancy and 27 cases mentioned as premature. This gives an overall prenatal mortality of 54°/oo, a figure that is only slightly higher than the figures found in Europe and the U.S.A. before 1945, where data between 40 and 50°/oo were registered in countries that nowadays have a perinatal mortality below 10°/oo.

5. Multiple pregnancies

In the notebook 70 twin births and two triplet births are mentioned. Both triplets are also considered in the memoirs (see 161 and 2292). From the 70 twins we find 15 cases mentioned in the memoirs (see Table of Families, herefore). Once again, Vrouw Schrader obviously used her memoirs to tell about extraordinary occurrences.

The frequency of multiple pregnancies (72 in $3060 = 2.35\%$) is high. It is probable that at the turn of the 18th century the frequency of twin pregnancies has been higher than at present by the higher number of multiparae, but a percentage of more than 2% indicates once more a concentration of pathology in the practice of Schrader.

Maternal mortality in 72 multiple pregnancies amounted to three (4%), (one case is mentioned in the memoirs, see 35); whereas the overall maternal mortality in single pregnancies amounted to around 0.6%. Perinatal mortality of the 146 children was 22%, of the single born children 4.5%.

The very pathological character of multiple pregnancy is apparent from these figures. At the same time these figures show the reliability of the data given by Vrouw Schrader. That the perinatal mortality, comparing the figures of Schrader with the present-day figure, shows a greater improvement for twins than for single children shows that the great improvement in present-day obstetrics is mainly reached in the field of pathology. The far better results reached nowadays in the treatment of placenta praevia are another example.

6. Artificial deliveries

If Vrouw Schrader had to interfere, this was mostly done by manual manoeuvres. A combination of external and internal procedures was often used. Often the woman was placed in (what we now call) steep Trendelenburg position or helped from behind, the head of the woman resting in the lap of another woman.

The total number of extractions (including versions and extractions) comes to 88 ($= 2.9\%$). These manipulations were done with much care and sometimes took much time. The very low number of uterine rupture (in all probability less than one or two percent in these very difficult labours) shows the dexterity and experience of Vrouw Schrader.

Instrumental deliveries were exceptional. In six cases Vrouw Schrader applied the instrument (the crotchet) herself. All are mentioned in the memoirs (see 74, 872, 968, 1485, 1810 and 2183). In ten cases she asked a man-midwife to perform this procedure (see the memoirs, cases 16, 74, 153, 2047 and 2594, and the notebook, cases 319, 484, 662, 2131 and 3052). As in case 74 the midwife and the man-midwife both applied a crotchet, there are in all 15 cases in which an instrument was used (0.5%). In this series of 15 horrible deliveries all children were stillborn (in fact all children were already dead before the operation started) and four mothers (see 16, 153, 2594, 3052) died as well. This gives a maternal mortality of four in 15. If we add the 15 cases of instrumental deliveries to the 88 deliveries with manual manipulation then we come to a total number of 103 artificial births (= 3%).

7. Manual removal of the placenta

The man-midwives and surgeons of the 17th and 18th century advocated an aggressive attitude towards the placenta. They feared that the womb would close itself after the birth of the child, making a removal of the placenta impossible. In 1701, Van Deventer defended an aggressive attitude with the following arguments:[8]
1) immediately after birth of the child it is easy to bring in the hand or even the whole arm and it is less painful;
2) if you wait and lose time with conservative methods (for example methods to let the woman vomit or to induce a coughing-fit or to let her blow) than it can be too late, since the womb will close itself;
3) if there is a partial inversio uteri you can redress it immediately;
4) labour is ended in a shorter time, and
5) sometimes you discover a second child.
Even after a spontaneous birth of the placenta he thinks it better to bring the hand into the uterus. Sometimes there is a second child, sometimes a part of the placenta is still left behind and sometimes a partial inversion of the womb has to be redressed.

The same attitude was advocated by Cornelis Kelderman (1697).[9] Vrouw Schrader did not follow this aggressive attitude. In her notebook we could find 64 cases of manual removal of the placenta (2%). As many of these cases were in combination with an artificial delivery of the child we can conclude that in all 3060 deliveries mentioned in the notebook in about 4% some sort of interference by manual manipulations has taken place, whereas in more than 95% the birth process was spontaneous.

8. Congenital malformations

Occasionally Vrouw Schrader mentions congenital malformations, but most likely only if there was a very serious one. It is improbable that in more than 3100 newborn children only one case of clubfoot could be registered (notebook, case 1128). The same holds true for harelip and palatoschisis. Three (see 89, 1533? and 2431; all in the memoirs) seems rather a low number.

Anencephaly can be diagnosed in case 2047 and perhaps in 2075. Hydrocephaly seems probable in 2239 (notebook) and 2431; spina bifida in 1286 (notebook) and in 2686; and a myelomeningocele with microcephaly in 2771. Hernia funiculi umbilicalis is described in case 1672, 1847 and 2885 (notebook). A case of chondrodystrophia can be assumed in 2933, but sometimes it is very difficult to interpret her description (as in case 69 in the notebook).

Like almost everybody in these times Vrouw Schrader believed strongly in the possibility that strong emotions or intensively looking at something during pregnancy could cause deformities in the expected child ("verzien"). Such explanations of severe malformations are given in 1633, 1672, 2075 and 2771, all mentioned in the memoirs, and in 1241 (only mentioned in the notebook).

9. Family analysis

A very interesting possibility to get more information from the notebook is collecting all cases in which Vrouw Schrader assisted in consecutive deliveries of the same woman. A few examples collected by Van Lieburg, are given here.[10]

A. In all Vrouw Schrader assisted 13 times in deliveries of Gritie, wife of cord maker Johannes. Only one case is mentioned in the memoirs (see 1062). The first delivery took place in 1699, the 13th in 1712. The results were as follows:

I) 1699 Spontaneous birth of a boy. All well (see 433).
II) 1701 Spontaneous birth. A boy. All well (see 675).
III) 1704 Spontaneous birth. A girl. All well (see 955).
IV) 1704 Very difficult breech extraction. A boy. Died after one hour (see 106?).
V) 1705 Spontaneous abortion (see 1140).
VI) 1706 Premature labour (about seven months). Spontaneous. A boy. Died after two hours (see 1249).
VII) 1707 Premature, spontaneous birth (about seven months). A girl. Died after one hour (see 1347).
VIII) 1707 Very premature spontaneous birth (about five months). Sex of child not mentioned (see 1401).
IX) 1708 Premature, spontaneous birth (about seven months). A girl (see 1489).
X) 1709 Premature, spontaneous. Sex unknown. Dead after one hour (see 1610).
XI) 1710 Abortion about 18 weeks. Stillborn. Much amniotic fluid (see 1758).

XII) 1711 Spontaneous, premature (about seven months). Girl. Stillborn (see 1835).

XIII) 1712 Premature (about 22 weeks). A boy. Died (see 1918).

After three normal spontaneous deliveries of healthy children a very difficult breech extraction took place. The child died after one hour. Thereafter, eight pregnancies all ended prematurely. The first two pregnancies and the tenth with live born children, who died after one to two hours, all other children were stillborn. We can think of two explanations for this "historia morbi". The first and by far most probable is a Rhesus-sensibilisation in which the homozygous Rhesuspositive husband via his children sensitized his Rhesusnegative wife. The difficult breech extraction can have given rise to a fetal-maternal transfusion. In accordance with this supposition is, that the results of the consecutive pregnancies became worse and worse. (This rules out syphilis as a possibility, for then we had expected a gradual improvement.) Also the fact that at least in one pregnancy (XI) is mentioned there was a great amount of amniotic fluid supports our hypothesis.

The other explanation could be: incompetence of the cervix caused by the difficult breech extraction. This could explain the early births thereafter, but than we expect the birth of live born children; very often sudden and almost painless. It could not explain hydramnios. Neither the decrease in duration of pregnancy in consecutive births, nor the fact that many children were stillborn. This history must have been a riddle in the times of Vrouw Schrader. It took more than two centuries before an explanation could be given.

B. As an example of a "good breeder" we can give the history of Rinke, wife of Jackop Dronrip. None of these deliveries were worthwhile to be mentioned in the memoirs!

I) 1700 Normal labour, healthy child (were not married) (see notebook 526).

II) 1703 Normal labour, healthy child. Married (see 878).

III) 1706 Normal labour, healthy child (see 1129).

IV) 1706 Normal labour, healthy child (see 1260).

V) 1708 Normal labour, healthy child (see 1462).

VI) 1711 Twins, both girls in complete breech presentation (see 1790).

C. In the memoirs, a concentration of pathology, we find examples of "bad breeders" like Gritie, wife of Sybele, smith. Only the second case (643) is mentioned in the memoirs.

I) 1699 Prolonged labour. Lasted more than two days. Child died at least two days before birth (see 393).

II) 1701 Early spontaneous rupture of the membranes. Head presentation with prolapse of one arm (see 643). Version and very difficult extraction of the dead child. After three days the mother died (infection?, incomplete rupture of the uterus?)

D. Another example is Trintie, wife of the Mayor Synya.
I) 1722 In pregnancy constant loss of blood for three months. At 20 weeks abortion (see notebook 2059).
II) 1724 Early spontaneous rupture of the membranes. After several days a quick and spontaneous delivery of a healthy girl (see notebook 2097).
III) 1727 Early spontaneous rupture of the membranes. Transverse position of the child. Prolapse of the cord. Difficult version and extraction. Child died during labour. Mother well. This last case is mentioned in the memoirs (see memoirs 2265).

Undoubtedly further analysis of all cases will bring more interesting facts and connections. We hope to publish more about this very interesting and unique notebook in the near future.

NOTES

1. L. Bourgeois, *Observations diverses, sur la stérilité, perte de faecondité fruict, accouchements et maladies des femmes et enfants nouveaunaiz, amplement traictées et heureusement practiquées*, Paris 1626.
2. C. Solingen, *Spiegel der Vroed-vrouwen door Justina Dittrichs, genaemt Siegemund*, Amsterdam: Jan ten Hoorn, 1691.
3. Jane Sharp, *The midwives book or the whole art of midwifery discovered*, London 1671.
4. See the Dutch edition, cases 101, 1988, 2187, 2201, 2394, 2738, 2998, 3052.
5. See the Dutch edition, case 1465, 2132, 2979, 2980 and 3027, and in all probability, also in 759, 971 and 2462.
6. F. Mauriceau, *Observations sur la grossesse et l'accouchements des femmes etc.*, Paris 1694 (4th edition).
7. Thomas E. Cone, "De pondere infantum recens natorum", *Pediatrics* 25 (1961) 480-498.
8. H. van Deventer, *Manuale Operatien, zijnde een Nieuw Ligt voor Vroed-meesters en Vroed-vrouwen*, Den Haag 1701.
9. C. Kelderman, *Ampt ende Plicht der Vroed-vrouwen*, Alphen a/d Rijn: Stafleu, 1981 (Librije der Geneeskonst, 7).
10. The demographical research has been executed by F.A. van Lieburg.

1722

den eersten April vor een sagte banker   325
't porgasien niet eet temper poeder gemaekt om
het blaet te sueren vor hat grotte ebelke   0 — 16

1722 den 5 Augustus nae diesens gesonden vor sacker
Louwrick syn huyse dij haer quaelick in haer
lyem gestelt waer ... velder hande dyester;
en mesters gemedi ... hat hat ... en baatjen
noch haer een ... lijster op het lijf
gesonden --
Een pott ... dringende pijsen en sallue ... 10
Vor pijsers suoerserum   0 — 16
dr ij ... om in jeneuer te doen vor open lijf — 6
                                              2 — 4

724 den 3 Juny ij wijtze Tammes dochter van
Rijkerd bij mij gekomen datse 5 weeken ouwt in de
Creim vroeu en sedert dij tit ser ellendig in haar
lyam datse nit allg met sin konde ... en ook
een duster in haar lijst met gedurige ... maeg
nit op syn platz waer gebracht
haer gevisentert verbonden met een steuringe ... f — 4
en boijer in geyeuen auens ——   0 — 4
den 4 dito weer een heijs en verbant ——   0 — 3
ook een pijer in geyeuen ——   0 — 4
ook en pott sallue ——   0 — 6
ook en porgasie ——   0 — 6

Page from the Notebook of Vrouw Schrader (folio 325)

Hilary Marland
AN INTRODUCTION TO THE MEMOIRS OF VROUW SCHRADER

The memoirs of Catharina Geertruida Schrader give a case-by-case description of a selection of the deliveries which she attended during her many years in practice as a midwife in Friesland in The Netherlands during the final years of the 17th and first half of the 18th centuries. The memoirs are based on the notebook which was kept by Vrouw Schrader between 1693 and 1745, and deal predominantly with the more complicated cases which she encountered during this period. Schrader's notebook and memoirs were apparently meant to serve as a personal record of her midwifery practice, and as a tribute to God for the support He had rendered her in her calling. They were also, as she writes at the conclusion of her memoirs, intended to serve as a guide to her successors in the practice of midwifery.

The notebook and memoirs of Catharina Schrader are of interest to those concerned with the history of midwifery practice and obstetrics on many counts. Diaries of the sort written by Vrouw Schrader, if not unique, are at least very rare, especially for such an early period. Schrader's notebook covers a long, almost unbroken, time span *and* records a large number of cases, 3060 in number, many being written up in some detail. Other known and extant midwives' diaries are rarities, and those that do survive are generally records of a rather later period, such as the two American journals, of Susanna Müller of Providence Township, Pennsylvania (1791-1815), and Martha Moore Ballard of Augusta, Maine (1785-1812), both of which cover the late 18th and early 19th centuries, and much shorter periods than Schrader's notebook.[1] Ballard's diary is considered as being one of the most important sources for the study of colonial midwifery. But while elaborating on the social aspects of childbirth and giving some indication of the work of early American midwives, the journal does not give details of the cases which Mrs Ballard attended, even when these were complicated or, in Ballard's terminology, "supernatural" deliveries.[2]

Such evidence as we have on the activities of midwives in Europe and America during the 17th and 18th centuries suggests that the norm was for their case loads to be low, although the epitaph of Elizabeth Phillips, whose death in 1761 brought to an end her more than forty-year career as a New England midwife, claimed that she "...by ye blessing of God,...

brought into this world above three thousand children".[3] Adrian Wilson has suggested that most English midwives during the late 17th and early 18th centuries experienced low levels of practice. For example, in early 18th-century Norwich midwives saw on average only 55 cases per annum.[4] The evidence of Elizabeth Cellier, the prominent London midwife and advocate of a college of midwives, suggests that during the 1680s there were between 1000 and 2000 midwives practising in London,[5] each seeing only between eight and seventeen births a year. Low levels of practise precluded the development of technical competence, and it seems that most midwives would have had little knowledge or skill concerning complicated cases. Catharina Schrader's practice, therefore, was probably outstanding, not only because of her high case load, in many years more than one hundred cases, but also because so many of the cases which she attended were far from straightforward. Not only is Schrader's notebook a rare source, but the exceptional nature of her practice lends it more than usual interest for the historian.

Within the confines of this project, it has proved impossible to translate Schrader's notebook in its entirety. Out of the 3060 deliveries recorded by Vrouw Schrader, 894 (29 per cent) of the cases, gynaecologically the most interesting and exceptional, were transcribed in the original Dutch edition of the notebook, published in 1984.[6] Out of the notebook entries, 122 cases were chosen by Schrader for her collection of memoirs (see table 1). The memoirs, representing the cases which Vrouw Schrader herself regarded as being the most remarkable and significant, have been selected for translation into English. The cases included in Vrouw Schrader's memoirs were not necessarily typical of those which she dealt with in her day-to-day practice. Rather, they are composed of the more complicated cases which she encountered malpresentations, labours of excessive duration, deliveries complicated by the age, deformity or sickness of the mother, or malformation of the child, and cases botched, in Schrader's estimation, by other midwives. The cases presented in the memoirs were described in much greater detail by Schrader than the more straightforward deliveries contained in the notebook.

Vrouw Schrader's notebook and memoirs give us a close insight into the role of a midwife, albeit not a typical one, in the birth process, describing her obstetric procedures in some detail. While by no means approaching the degree of meddlesomeness as described by Edward Shorter "Constantly tugging and hauling at the mother's birth canal, at the infant's head, and at the placenta, they were captives of a folkloric view that the best midwife is the one who interferes most",[7] Schrader does not fulfill the "golden age" picture of midwife-attended confinements, such as that offered by Catherine Scholten "In all circumstances the midwife's chief duty was to comfort the woman in labor while they both waited on nature".[8] Vrouw Schrader impresses us in her memoirs as being an "interventionalist", and not only in a strictly technical sense. In the cases Schrader describes she apparently viewed herself as the prime mover and active party in the delivery scene. Instruments were used rarely, in cases of extreme exigency, almost without exception only when the child was already dead, and usually only after a surgeon or man-midwife had been summoned to the delivery. But Schrader was a busy manipulator, dilating the cervix, stretching the passages, referring often to the fact that she "had to make all the openings", employing a variety of birth positions, pulling the child out with "great force", and frequently practising podalic version, her instinct and experience leading her to prefer to deliver the child feet first. She was also extremely anxious to quickly relieve the parturient woman of the afterbirth.

It should be re-emphasised that many of the cases described in Schrader's memoirs were complicated and dangerous, often for both mother and child (or children), and as such not representative of the vast majority of deliveries, which needed no intervention from a midwife or any other birth attendant. Schrader was frequently fetched to the delivery scene when other midwives had already given up the case, often days after the confinement had commenced. Schrader was very much a midwife of her times, when a high level of, essentially manual, intervention was standard, in both complicated *and* normal deliveries,[9] and when much ignorance still prevailed concerning conception, pregnancy and female anatomy.[10] This level of intervention was perhaps in part at least a response to the constant fear of death or illness which was linked to maternity; a skillful or inventive midwife could be seen as actively tackling, "engaging in battle", these very real dangers. Death was a frequent accompaniment of pregnancy and childbirth for the mother,[11] child or both. Bearing children, especially if complications set in, could be terrifying, dangerous and fatal. "For ought you to know your Death has entered into you, you may have conceived that which determines but about Nine Months more at the most, for you to live in the World."[12] Women were worn out and prematurely aged by a continuing series of pregnancies, miscarriages, often mishandled deliveries, nursing and the not infrequent bereavement linked to the death of a child. All too often this cycle was aggravated by poverty and want.[13] Fear of death was coupled with the dread of being maimed for life. Postpartum complications, vesico-vaginal and recto-vaginal fistulas, perineal tears, prolapsed uterus and infection, could force women into invalidism for the rest of their lives or result in constant and extreme embarrassment and discomfort.[14]

Atypical or not, the deliveries described in Vrouw Schrader's notebook provide a sobering account of women's experiences in childbirth, with case after case of suffering, pain, permanent injury to mother and child, and death. It was not without good reason that Schrader entitled her notebook *Memoryboeck van de Vrouwens* (Memoirs of the Women), dedicating it to the women she had delivered.

The memoirs were written when Schrader, retired from her midwifery practice, was already in her mid-eighties. Given this, the enormous time span between some of the cases taking place and being re-written in the memoirs, and Vrouw Schrader's tendency to embellish and exaggerate rather than the reverse, the original notebook extracts frequently differ from the memoirs, sometimes in emphasis, but often also in the facts given. Where this has occurred details of the notebook entry are given in parenthesis following the relevant case. Any additional information taken from the notebook has also been presented in this way.

An attempt has been made to retain something of Schrader's style and the atmosphere which she created in the translation of the memoirs. The task of translating the memoirs was far from straightforward, not least because of Schrader's usage of a mixture of Dutch, German and Frisian, complicated by her own unique and varied spelling, non-existent punctuation and erratic sentence construction, and enlivened by her very individualistic expressions. An effort has been made to be accurate, but at the same time also to retain the flavour of Schrader's descriptions and language; in effect, to produce a translation of the memoirs which an English-speaking contemporary of Schrader might have written. For the sake of readability and consistency, and to avoid "historical quaintness", the text has not been translated into "18th-century English", and spelling, capitalization and punctuation have been modernized.

NOTES

1. "Susanna Müller, 1756-1815. An Old German Midwife's Record", ed. by M.D. Learned and C.F. Bride (n.p., n.d.). Located at Library of the College of Physicians of Philadelphia; Charles E. Nash, *The History of Augusta: First Settlements and Early Days as A Town Including the Diary of Mrs. Martha Moore Ballard* (Augusta, Me., 1904). Both cited in Judy Barrett Litoff, *American Midwives 1860 to the Present* (Westport, Conn. and London: Greenwood Press, 1978) 6.
2. For details of Mrs Ballard's midwifery practice and diary, see Jane B. Donegan, "'Safe Delivered', but by Whom? Midwives and Men-Midwives in Early America", in: Judith Walzer Leavitt (ed.), *Women and Health in America* (Madison, Wisconsin: University of Wisconsin Press, 1984) 308-309 and Richard W. Wertz and Dorothy C. Wertz, *Lying-In. A History of Childbirth in America* (New York: Schocken, 1979) 9-11.

3. Quoted in Francis R. Packard, *History of Medicine in the United States* (New York: Hafner, 1931), vol. I, 49.
4. Adrian Wilson, *Childbirth in Seventeenth- and Eighteenth-Century England*, unpublished PhD thesis (University of Sussex, 1982) 120.
5. J.H. Aveling, *English Midwives* (London: J. & A. Churchill, 1872; reprinted New York: AMS Press, 1977) 77. Cited ibidem, 123.
6. M.J. van Lieburg (ed), *C.G. Schrader's Memoryboeck van de Vrouwens. Het notitieboek van een Friese vroedvrouw 1693-1745 (with an obstetric commentary by Prof.Dr. G.J. Kloosterman)* (Amsterdam: Editions Rodopi, 1984) For a review of the Dutch edition of the notebook, see Willem Frijhoff, "Vrouw Schraders beroeps-journaal: Overwegingen bij een publikatie over arbeidspraktijk in het verleden", *Tijdschr. Gesch. Geneesk. Natuurw. Wisk. Techn.* 8 (1985) 27-38.
7. Edward Shorter, *A History of Women's Bodies*, New York: Basic Books, 1982.
8. Catherine M. Scholten, "'On the Importance of the Obstetrick Art': Changing Customs of Childbirth in America, 1760-1825", in: Judith Walzer Leavitt (ed.), *Women and Health in America*, 144.
9. Irvine Loudon cites the period between 1700 and 1780 as one of high levels of intervention in normal and lingering births, prior to 1733 being mainly of a manual nature and after 1733, following the publication of the design of the forceps, both manual and instrumental. Irvine Loudon, "Nature versus Intervention in Obstetrics: An Historical Survey", paper given at Wellcome Unit, Oxford, 1 May, 1986 in the Graduate Seminar series.
10. For the development of obstetrics and gynaecology between the 16th and 18th centuries and ideas concerning sexuality, menstruation, conception, pregnancy and childbirth, see Audrey Eccles, *Obstetrics and Gynaecology in Tudor and Stuart England*, London: Croom Helm, 1982.
11. For maternal mortality see, for example, B.M. Willmott Dobbie, "An attempt to estimate the true rate of maternal mortality, sixteenth to eighteenth centuries", *Medical History* 26 (1982) 79-90; Audrey Eccles, "Obstetrics in the 17th and 18th Centuries and its implications for Maternal and Infant Mortality", *Bull. Soc. soc. Hist. Med.* 20 (June, 1977) 8-11; and Irvine Loudon, "Deaths in childbed from the eighteenth century to 1935", *Medical History* 30 (1986) 1-41.
12. Cotton Mather, *Elizabeth in Her Holy Retirement: An Essay to Prepare a Pious Woman for Her Lying-in; or, Maxims and Methods of Piety, to Direct and Support an Hand Maid of the Lord, Who Expects a Time of Travail* (Boston, 1710) 3. Quoted in: Catherine M. Scholten, "On the Importance of the Obstetrick Art", 143.
13. See Mireille Laget, "Childbirth in Seventeenth- and Eighteenth- Century France: Obstetrical Practices and Collective Attitudes", in: Robert Forster and Orest Ranum (eds), *Medicine and Society in France. Selections from the Annales*, vol. 6 (Baltimore and London: Johns Hopkins University Press, 1980), especially pp. 146-157 and 167-173, for a sobering account of the pain and suffering surrounding childbirth in Ancien Regime France.
14. See also Judith Walzer Leavitt, *Brought to Bed. Childbearing in America 1750-1950* (New York and Oxford: Oxford University Press, 1986), especially chapter 1, for the fear of death surrounding pregnancy and birth, maternal mortality rates and the injuries.

1693 februarÿ

1693 op vastelavent avens ben jck vor de aller
Erste Reÿs van mÿn Leven tot wÿns gehalt bÿ een
Wedeuw haar man Chles Jansen genamt in een schricke
onweer storm wint harde vorst dar raeckten
wÿ vert met ens drÿen nede slede int ÿs men konde
niet sten van weegen de wint den staeken mÿ de
Jaeken ÿs en mÿn beesten dat mÿ het blaut in de
keusen lip en quamen met de slede tÿndelick to
wÿns Suren gang bÿ nae doot sÿnde men droÿ
mÿ int hus en braeken nÿ de mont epen goeten
nÿ brandewin in de ment dar was een goet fur
ontbÿde do wat, Eÿsse ses. Een bavse met snee
En freef dar nede kannden so lange dat er leven
gwam anders hade jck all mÿn leven bedorven
geweft den weer bekomen wat weesende fouw ock
te vrouw geholpen weesen en alis o haar ouit
man broders het alles ontnomen haden en gefeÿt
feÿ feuw nit Craamen fo war andes kindes tÿm
veel gelegen dar doch altit vel ant leven, en vrouw
hade en seer swaare baaringe gelietse in haar vÿf
Craamen ock geweft wat desse demael z van
Luwarder vrout vrauwen gehat hade jck au bur te
steure en hÿ verhorde nÿ en verlefte de vrouw te
grots weÿse van haar en meÿ van ven en bren
dochter dese in Leÿtinge vor de Erste n aut
waar benaint de Heere sÿ gedanckt alles well en
de vrouw kreÿ en haar goet wer

THE MEMOIRS OF VROUW SCHRADER
Translated and annotated by Hilary Marland

Thereupon in my eighty-forth year of old age in my empty hours I sat and thought over what miracles The Lord had performed through my hands to unfortunate, distressed women in childbirth. So I decided to take up the pen in order to refresh once more my memory, to glorify and make great God Almighty for his great miracles bestowed on me. Not me, but You oh Lord be the honour, the glory till eternity. And also in order to alert my descendants so that they can still become educated. And I have pulled together the rare occurrences from my notes.

In my thirty-eight years living in Hallum in Friesland I saw my good, learned and highly esteemed, and by God and the people loved husband, go to his God to the great sadness of me and the inhabitants, leaving six small children in my thirty-eight years of age. But then it pleased God to choose me for this important work: by force almost through good doctors and the townspeople because I was at first struggling against this, because it was such a weighty affair. Also I thought that it was for me and my friends below my dignity; but finally I had myself won over. This was also The Lord's wish.

1.   1693 on 9 January fetched to Jan Wobes's wife, Pittie, in Hallum.[1] A very heavy labour. Came with his face upwards. A dangerous birth for the child and very difficult for me. The afterbirth had to be pulled loose.[2] But everything well. (The notebook mentions that Schrader was called at five o'clock in the morning to the labour. With God's "grace and help",[3] Schrader delivered a boy.)[4]

3.   1693 on Shrove Tuesday (26 February) in the evening I was fetched for the very first journey in my life to Wijns to a widow whose husband was called Chlas Jansen, in terrible weather, stormy wind, hard frost.[5] The three of us travelled by sleigh over the ice. The wind blew so hard that one could not stand. Pieces of ice got stuck in my legs, so that blood dripped into my hose. And came at last by sleigh to Wijns, three hours going;[6] we were almost dead. The people carried me into the house and forced my mouth open; and poured brandy into my mouth. There was a good fire. I thawed out a little. First I demanded a bowl with snow and rubbed my hands and feet with it until life came into them. Otherwise I would have been

ruined for life. After I recovered again, I went to help the woman. And also her dead husband's brothers had taken everything away from her and had said that she would not give birth; therefore the life of this child was of great consequence. The woman had a very heavy labour, like her previous labours had also been; she had had two midwives from Leeuwarden [in her previous labours].[7] I prayed to [The] Lord, and he answered me and delivered the woman of a good, big daughter to the great delight of her and me. This introduction was oppressive[8] for the first time. The Lord be thanked. All well. And the woman got all her belongings back.

16.   1693 on 2 November I was fetched to Marrum to Hincke, the wife of Bauwke Binders, merchant. Was there a day and a night. Did everything that art required.[9] It seemed an uncomplicated birth. And I wanted to deliver her by art, but because I still had little experience, I wished to have a surgeon[10] with me to avoid all scandal.[11] But they let another midwife be called.[12] When she [the other midwife] came to her she said she would deliver her immediately. And I was rejected completely [sent away]. The women tortured the labouring woman for two days, so I eventually said, she would never deliver her. And I did not want to involve myself again. And I said to the midwife that she should let her be and not torment her anymore. She gave completely wrong information and said that the child now lay with his shoulder forward, first with his back [presenting]. I investigated and found that it [the child] had not moved a hand's breadth compared with when I was attending the day before. It was the wrong way round.[13] I said, that a man-midwife, doctor (Theodorus) Winnter, had to be called immediately from Leeuwarden.[14] When he came he inquired first of me how it was with the women in labour, as I had been the first to be with her. Then he questioned the other [midwife]. Then he went to the woman in labour, investigated the case and said, we could not help her. Removed the dead child with an instrument (hook),[15] but the woman worsened on the third day, got looseness and died. The doctor ridiculed the other midwife; gave me great repute. Gave me a solemn testimonial and great honour. (The notebook entry maintains that Schrader was present at the labour two whole days.[16] She tried to get an experienced surgeon, who did come, but then excused himself before the second midwife was called. Schrader had predicted that the child was already dead.)

18.   1693 on 24 December I was fetched to De Leie to the wife of a horseman, whose mother was a midwife. And [the mother] had tortured her two days and nights. The child lay very squashed. The

woman and I had a hard time. And with The Lord's blessing, I helped her in half an hour. All well for mother and child. (The notebook gives a different date, 31 December. Schrader was called in the evening, and delivered the woman of a daughter. Here she claims that she helped her in an hour.)

20.   1694 on 27 January I was fetched to the wife of Derck Jans, Antie, after another [midwife] had been with her two days and nights. Everything was in a terrible state. The child was deeply embedded, with the feet round the neck [and] trapped behind the pubic bone, the cord round the legs and round the neck. Must be choked. Was stuck two hours in the birth canal. Had to loosen it with enormous difficulty. I had almost given up, but The Lord brought solution. The mother does well. (The notebook mentions that she was fetched on Sunday morning. The child was dead.)

35a.[17] 1694 on 6 October fetched to Nes on Ameland[18] to a skipper's wife. Had been in labour five days. [They] could not loosen her from the afterbirth. After that I was fetched to Hallum, but as soon as I came there she [the woman in labour] said, woman, you've come too late. And she closed her eyes and died. Had I been earlier, I think I could have saved the mother and child.

35b.   1694 on 6 October summoned to Ameland to the wife of a skipper of a big ship. Had been in labour five days with twins. The first one was born alive, the second was born dead two days later. And the afterbirth remained behind. And then I still had to be fetched over the sea. When I came indoors, she sat up [and] said to me, woman you've come too late. With that she died immediately, which was a great shock for me. Oh poor martyrs, who come under such torment from midwives.

39.   1695 on 16 December I went to de Nieuwe Zijl to Teirck Pitter's wife, Hanntie. The water was already gone [broken] when I came to her. Found the child very squashed and sideways before the birth canal. With much work I finally got it with its feet first before the birth canal.[19] But I succeeded. The second child came [presented] sideways. I had very great difficulty before I got it by its feet. Then the birth canal closed round its neck, and had to remain like this;[20] however the mother and one child is saved. This was my last case in these places. And then I went to Dokkum.[21] (The notebook states that it took from morning to evening before it was all over. This was a terribly heavy case.)

54.   1696 on 12 March I was fetched to the skipper Bonteko's wife, Barber. The waters were already expanded, but I couldn't observe the child till the waters broke, which were very clouded and thick.

Then the bottom presented, shortly after the shoulder, and side. With great difficulty I got its feet. Its chin got stuck on the pubic bone [ijsbeen]. While it was hard work for me, with the help of my God all was well for mother and child. (The notebook adds that the neck of the womb closed around the child's neck: "Oh Lord, save me from such unfortunate births".)

72. 1696 on Tuesday, 22 July [=June] I was fetched to Janke, the wife of Zitze Jouwes, who is a wagon maker. And with the help of my God, without which it would have been impossible, delivered her of a son. It was a very heavy [labour]. The child lay on its side, turned very awkwardly. Finally with much force and trouble I got its feet. In the presence of a man-midwife and our minister, who gave me great praise. Everything still well for mother and child. Oh God, You be honoured and thanked. (The notebook entry added that it was very difficult because vicar Schregardus was there, together with doctor Pitter Vanij.)

74. 1696 on 13 July I was fetched to the carpenter's wife, Bauwkie Frerick Ydes, whose waters had broken [while she was] at Leeuwarden, at her mothers. [She] went by towboat[22] and came to Dokkum.[23] Because it was a bad situation, I was fetched. The womb was closed around its [the child's] neck, with the navel string around the child's neck. It took four days, and was terribly heavy work. I gave up. Then they got another [midwife], who said it would be over quickly. She sat a day and a night with the cloths on her lap. She was a pupil. I made sure that surgeon Pitter came. He worked with the woman till he was worn out. Finally, with no other alternative, we used an instrument. And the surgeon didn't want to be without me for a moment. Together we fetched the dead child out with a hook each. And the mother had a healthy childbed.[24] And after that still had more children, and lived for forty more years. Oh Lord, save all people. (The notebook claims that the woman was in labour for three days. The navel string was wrapped three times around the child's neck. The mother was healthy after the delivery.)

88. 1696 on 17 August fetched to Maryken, wife of Jackopus, a cord maker. Delivered two daughters. One was lying [...?], while the first came awkwardly with the shoulders [presenting]. Had to get hold of the feet with great difficulty. But managed it. The afterbirth was grown in. But all was well. (All was well for mother and child[ren?]. The notebook adds that Schrader had to pull the afterbirth out.)

89. On 18 August 1696 with wife of Cornelis Jan, tile maker, Aryantie. Had a very heavy birth. The child lay squashed in the side. I had to

pull the afterbirth loose. The child had a harelip. (The notebook informs us that this case was in Oostersingel. The child was a girl. Schrader stresses she had to do a "terrible lot" with the afterbirth till it could be loosened.)

150. On 6 May 1697 fetched to Auwkie, the wife of the miller, Jan Berens. And delivered her of children, which were lying in a very queer way. Had to disentangle them both inside and pull them with their feet. Had much difficulty with the afterbirth. Everything still well for mother and child[ren?]. (The notebook mentions that the case was in the Aalsumerpoort[25]. Schrader delivered two daughters. The first presented with her bottom, the other with her feet. Praises God: "He saves me from accidents.")

153. 1697 on 17 May I went to Schuwkye, wife of Johanes Wytzes, innkeeper, who had danced on the previous days with a young man, supposedly from Kanck, so that he could no longer keep up with her. For this The Lord punished her, because she made her pregnant body suffer so much. She had three days of terrible labour. Very closed tight. The child was stuck, so she had to be delivered through art. The people fetched surgeon Pitter, who was working on her for a whole day, with the greatest difficulty in the world, so that he fainted away three times. But finally he and I got the child out together with a hook each. And the woman remained stable for three days. Then got heavy looseness and has died. (The notebook informs us that the case was in Aalsum, near Dokkum. It does not mention anything relating to dancing with a young man! Schrader was with the woman from Monday to Thursday. The child presented in a straightforward way. They had to pull the head out in pieces; the rest of the body was whole.)

161. 1697 on 30 June fetched to Oostrum to wife of Gerrben Teyepkes, farmer. There had already been another midwife there for two days. Could only help her with the first [child]. A dead child. But The Lord be thanked, I delivered her of the afterbirth within one hour. They both lay strangely. Turned them. The middle one was dead. The afterbirth was stuck, so that [there were] three children; one living, two dead. So that there were three children. They were big; the parents small, delicate people. The woman fresh and healthy. (The notebook states that the first child was dead, the second alive, and the third dead. Two boys and a girl, who was alive. There were three afterbirths. Schrader managed the deliveries in an hour. The smallest and last child presented with its bottom.)

219. 1696 on 28 December outside the Woudpoort with farmer Meyndert Dudes, after she had been tortured in heavy labour for two days by

a midwife. And [the other midwife] could not help her. When I came, I found that the child was stuck behind the pubic bone [ijsbeen]. Helped her in a quarter of an hour. All well. The Lord be thanked. (The notebook adds that the child was a daughter.)

282. 1698 on 3 July [to] Hincke, wife of Sibran Willems, baker, on the Vleesmarkt [meat market]. Found a big water with a badly turned child. I asked if she had labour pains. She said, no. I went home [and] said, as soon as you begin to feel the labour slightly, they must fetch me immediately. But the whole night, still half a night, nothing happened. The next day I went there in the afternoon and asked the woman if she still had not noticed any change. No. Thereupon I investigated the case. It was as before. I said, come, let us fetch friends and neighbours,[26] I must help you immediately. She, can we? So I had no labour pains. I, yes, let me just start, otherwise you and I might easily have a mishap. I went on, broke a big water. The child lay on its side. Turned it. Looked for the feet. Got it without pain or sorrow. Then another big water presented. The creature [child] came immediately. Turned it again, got the feet and delivered the woman immediately, without pain or anguish. A healthy childbed. A son and a daughter. They stayed long alive. God works in a mysterious way. (The notebook entry states that the woman was delivered of two sons. The second child came with the hand presenting, the first one came without difficulty.)

365. 1699 on 15 February fetched to Gebke, wife of the painter, Jackop Isebrant. Found that it [the child] lay with it shoulders forward. I broke the water. Turned it. Just managed with great trouble to get hold of the feet. It was a dangerous, heavy birth. The child was dead, the mother does well. (The notebook states that the child must have been suffocated.)

418. 1699 on 16 September to wife of soldier, Jan Geritz, Gatzke, a woollen worker. [Delivered] her of a son with heavy labour. A dead, heavy child. Had to fetch it from her with all force. The mother does well. But first could not hold her water. But improved by The Lord's goodness almost by its own accord. (The notebook adds that there was almost no hope naturally [for the child].)

420. 1699 on 24 September fetched to Clas Liewes Grittie, a linen worker, where a midwife, Saackie, had been busy with her for a whole day. But was not able to help her in a proper way. The child lay with his leg and a hand round the neck. The navel string outside the birth canal. I had to put her on her head in order to save her.[27] And got it in a quarter of an hour. But the child [was] dead, because the navel string hung outside the body.[28] The woman does well.

(The notebook entry reports that the other midwife had been trying to turn the child, but could not manage to do this. A hand and foot presented, the other foot was around the child's neck.)

423.   1699 on 4 October been called to Hilltie, wife of the town crier, Pitter Ludema. A heavy labour and very curious. Came repeatedly with his eyes before the birth canal. In the next moment in yet another presentation, then straight, then soon after awkwardly again. It was as if it [the child] flew in the body; such a birth has never come to me before. Moreover, the woman was very impatient. I had to put her on her head three times to turn it from behind. As soon as she was again in position, it was wrong again. I had to pull out the child from behind while leaning forward. Had almost not thought that the child could still be alive, but God's works are mysterious. The child and the mother are fresh and well. I gave it up, but they would not let me go. Locked the door and must [stay]. Oh Lord, save all people.

485.   1700 on 12 March I was fetched to Jackop Fittetie's wife. Found that there was no opening. It lay with its back before the birth canal. I fomented her underneath with a bath of "mother herbs"[29] to soften the parts and make it supple. Then turned it, but had to be born doubled up with [his] bottom [first]. Everything still well for mother and child. (The notebook adds that the child was almost dead, but improved later.)

486.   1700 on 13 March fetched to Oostersingel to Gebke, the wife of the painter and thread winder, Jackop Evers. Found that the water was gone. And his arms born,[30] the navel string outside. Turned it quickly and brought it forth. But it took a good hour using every device before one could bring him to life. But then everything well for the mother and child. It came from the navel string. (The notebook informs us that the child was a boy.)

521.   1700 18 July fetched to Rinsumageest to a labourer's wife. Was already in labour for the third day; another [midwife] was there. The child was stuck behind the pubic bone [ijsbeen]. Helped her immediately. (The notebook claims that the woman had been in labour for two days.)

525.   1700 on 30 July been to Tettie, the wife of a skipper, Liwe Douwes. It had been predicted by a doctor that she had two "vlygers"[31] in her, but I didn't reckon so. But she had no opening; so I fomented her with "mother herbs" in order to soften the passages. She was old in years. With God I helped her, so that she brought a living son into the world. But haven't come across any "vlygers".

581.   1701 on 27 January fetched to Akkerwoude to the widow of Simon

Gaabes, after she had been in labour for eight days. And found it
with its back in front of the birth canal. Looked for the feet. Turned
it. Had it immediately, to [the] great astonishment of all those who
were present. All well for mother and child.

595. 1701 on 1 March fetched to Broek, outside Dantumawoude, to the
blind midwife's daughter (Hynck). Found the navel string outside;
the child dead. The hand of the child presented. Turned it, got it by
the feet. It was hard work to say the least. Stayed with its head stuck
fast. Finally got it loose, but all still well for the mother.

597. 1701 on 4 March went to wife of Harmanus, wool-comber,
Catterina. The child lay with its back facing. Turned it. Got it by the
feet. Quickly. And happy for mother and child. (The notebook
informs us that the child was a girl.)

606. 1701 on 23 March to Hincke, the wife of the baker Lieuwe, who had
with her the midwife, Saekie, who had tormented the sufferer a long
time. I came [and] found the child lying with its stomach before the
birth canal, with both hands outside the birth canal. And the child
lay very squashed; could not get the feet. Had to put her over on her
head. With great difficulty got one foot, tied a string round it; then
got her back again in position [mother]. Then pulled towards me
[the string]. Then the hands went inside by themselves and held
[stayed in]. When I came the child was already dead. The afterbirth
[was] also very grown in. The mother does well. Oh very heavy
labour. (The notebook adds, "God save me from such terrible
deliveries".)

643. 1701 fetched outside the Hanspoort to Grittie, the wife of Jybele,
smith. Found the child lying very high. It lasted very long. Was no
opening there and the bones and muscles of the birth canal were
pinched very tight; therefore I fomented her. The child's head was
pressed flat by the great pressure. One arm came outside the birth
canal. Finally, I had to make a bad birth from a good one. Turned
it, looked for the feet and delivered a dead daughter. It was very
hard for the woman and I. The woman [was] saved. The Lord save
me and all people from such terrible occurrences. (The notebook
informs us that Schrader was fetched on 2 July. The waters had
broken early. The child could not be born, and the woman was
worn out. One arm hung outside the birth canal when the child was
dead. Dead after three days[?].)

661. 1701 I was fetched to Rynck Eckes's wife, who flooded a great deal
without labour. A doctor was fetched. She was also very watery and
flooded terribly. At last I was fetched again. The woman wrestled
with death. I said, she must deliver. Found the afterbirth loose

before the uterus. Then delivered her from it. Then the dead child lay sideways before the birth canal. Turned her. Delivered it [with] great difficulty. And she [the mother] died, very aware, in the presence of all her friends an hour after. She should have been delivered earlier with such heavy flooding. (The notebook mentions that the woman was called Hyllti. Her husband was a merchant. When Schrader arrived she found the woman worn out and at the end of a big flooding. Then at last she got her labour pains. After inspecting the case she found the afterbirth grown in at the front, which she had never heard of or come across before. She pulled it loose. Got the child by its feet. The mother died half an hour after.)

671. 1701 fetched to Driesum to a weaver's wife, after a previous midwife had delivered a baby the day before. Had to fetch her the day after again. Found that there was still another child, but could not help the woman with all her torturing. Went away [other midwife]. Then I was fetched. Found that the child [lay] with his stomach [first]. Turned it quickly. A living child. And [the] woman completely well. But the second day the woman was alone in the house; the people were milking. Then a strange man came in, who asked the woman in childbed whether he could light a tobacco pipe, which he did. After that the woman got such an attack of fits, that three men could not hold her. Together with periods without speech. Died the same day. One questioned if the person who had come in there had committed murder. The Lord knows best how. (The notebook adds that Schrader was fetched on 2 October. The other midwife had said at first that there was only one child. The second child lay with its chin behind the pubic bone [ijsbeen]. Schrader had to turn it from behind. The woman got a "pest-like" fever with periods without speech or reason.)

743. 1702 on 4 May [I] was fetched to Rinsumageest to the former sweetheart of the town clerk, Veenema, who had promised to be hers in marriage, but who had left her on the advice of friends. Was four days in labour. Could not be helped. Then I was fetched and delivered her quickly through the help of my God. Yet a heavy birth, because of the heartache caused to her. (The notebook mentions that she delivered a son. Another midwife had been there for three days. According to the baptismal register of Rinsumageest, the child was a daughter.)

796. 1702 on 12 October delivered two sons to the knitter, Swaantie. The first came well, the second with his stomach [first]. Had difficulty with turning [it]. Still all was well for mother and children. The Lord be praised and thanked.

825. 1703 on 24 January fetched to Dantumawoude to minister Bruning's first wife, Anna, where a midwife from Bergum had been there for two days.[32] Also two doctors and ministers. In her great necessity I was eventually also fetched. Found that the leg lay in front of the pubic bone [ijsbeen]. Solved that, but with great difficulty. It stuck there as if grown in fast. Still everything then well for mother and child.

852. 1703 in March (26) fetched to Hantum to a tailor's wife to pull the afterbirth loose, after she had been tormented a whole day by the midwife. Which, luckily, I managed immediately.

872. 1703 fetched outside the Woudpoort to Antie, the wife of Hottse, wagon maker. Lasted a day and night with terrible labour. Stuck fast and was dead. I gave it up, but they did not want to be without me. I tried all means, but could not win. But finally I had [to turn] to the instrument. I thrust the hook in the child's mouth and I got it. A big dead daughter. All is well. (The notebook states that the case took place on 3 June. The child was stuck with its shoulders on the pubic bone [ijsbeen]. Turned it so that the mouth was in front of the uterus. Schrader had put the woman on her head three times.)

968. 1704 on 10 March with the wife of Jan Teckes Osterbaan. Was two days in heavy labour. Could not deliver. A dead foetus was stuck. Had to get it with an instrument with great force. But all well for mother. (The notebook adds that it was a son.)

969. 1704 on 13 March I was fetched to Driesum to Gaabe Dudes's wife, Trintie, where the midwife had already delivered a daughter six hours before. She did not know what to do with the second [child]. I turned it, got it by the feet. A living son. So that she bore a son and a daughter. And all well.

971. 1704 on 13 March fetched to Joure to Schurt Douwes's wife, after a midwife from Ternaard had already been there for two days. [The other midwife] could not help the woman. The chin was behind the pubic bone [ijsbeen]. I helped her quickly, praise be, of a living son. (The notebook extract claims that the other midwife had been with the woman a whole night.)

1024. 1704 on 12 September fetched to Romkie, wife of Jorgen Sticker, butcher. And the water had already been gone [for] two days. She was already in her forties. But no opening. Had to make everything [for] her. I fomented her underneath with a herbal bath. With hardly any opening had to turn the child with difficulty. Delivered it with the feet. The second came in a good position half an hour after. All still well for mother and child[ren?]. (The notebook mentions that Schrader had to make room with her hands. She delivered two small girls.)

1030.   1704 on 20 September fetched to Rimke, wife of Jackop Fockeles, town-beadle, after she had been very sick for three days from [the] water. Have given her an enema twice. Got the first child successfully. Carried four pots of water away [from] under her. Delivered of two daughters. Everything still well.

1062.   1704 on 1 December been to Gritie, wife of cord maker, Johannes. Heavy labour, little opening. Got one leg; I had terrible difficulty with the other. Already had her on her head; could not get hold of it. A very heavy labour. And had almost given it up, but The Lord gave deliverance. Through The Lord's goodness all well for mother and child. (The notebook adds that one foot was behind pubic bone [ijsbeen]. Schrader put the woman twice on her head. A healthy son.)

1157.   1705 on 20 (25) October with a corporal's wife, Elske "kop of".[33] A dead child. Lay with its back before the birth canal. The water was already gone before I came. It lay very strangely. When I turned it, it stayed with its head in the birth canal. The string three times around its neck. I had to make it loose in pieces with the razor inside [the] body, before it could be born. (The notebook adds that it was terribly hard work to get the child. A dead daughter.)

1211.   The year 1706 on 9 (19) March fetched to Oosterwolde to Jackop Hemmes's wife, Sywke; there had been another midwife [there] for two days. Found that the womb was in front of the child's head and was shut very fast, which should have been put right earlier. The woman [other midwife] had no knowledge about it. And I had much difficulty to put it to rights, but soon all well for mother and child. A son.

1233.   1706 on 12 June fetched to Driesum to Berent, skipper. There was another [midwife] with her who had much tortured the woman. It was born with the head [first]. It was dead. And was stuck terribly fast. I had much to do there before I could get the dead child loose. Took me only a quarter of an hour to [the] great joy of the mother and others. The mother does well. (The notebook entry mentions that the labour had lasted a whole day before Schrader was called.)

1250.   1706 on 1 August been called to Lisken, wife of Pybe Jans, bricklayer, who had previously had four very big floodings. The fourth time. Examined her. Found the afterbirth grown in fast in front of the child. The woman was unconscious in a dead faint. I ordered that the woman must be delivered, but I wanted to have a doctor with me. She had no labour. The doctor said that he would administer something to induce labour. I said, that must not be, because the flood would become still heavier; I should deliver her

60

without labour. The doctor found this idea curious. I said, the child was dead. He insisted that it lived.[34] I pulled the afterbirth after I had loosened it on one side, looked for the feet and delivered it immediately to the shame of doctor Eysma, who stood firm that the child lived. And it was already completely rotten. The skin dropped off all over. That I could deliver her so without labour was occasioned because the parts became very slimy and tractable after such long-lasting flooding; otherwise this could not have occurred. And then the woman must be delivered without delay. Death is then close by. If I hadn't done this with this woman, she would not have lived another half hour; but she still has lived another thirty years after. She lay unconscious a day and a night. The doctor gave her a "heart strengthener" and got her strength back with time. In Dokkum. God alone be honoured. (The notebook extract states that the afterbirth was ingrown in front of the uterus. She got the afterbirth quickly and the flooding stopped little by little.)

1296. 1706 on 21 December fetched to Hantum to the wife of Gerit Meelis, after another midwife [had been there] three whole days and the Hantum surgeon, Nicklas. But with great difficulty I have with The Lord's help and assistance delivered the woman of a dead, rotten, big daughter to the great wonder of everyone. Everything through God's blessing upon me. The woman is well.

1374. 1707 on 3 September to Ymkie, wife of Johanes, potter. The child came with his knees before the birth canal. Pulled one foot to the birth canal; could not get the other one. Put her bending forward with the head down. Put her back again, got it immediately, but stayed with its head stuck fast. Had terribly much to do there. But got it still living, to [the] wonder of everyone who was there. The Lord be thanked. (The notebook adds that it was a girl.)

1382. 1707 on 15 September [went] to Margrita, wife of Auwke, gardener, after she had first had a heavy flooding. The child came first with one foot, then shortly after in another position of the body before the birth canal. Then came right again in front of the birth canal. And had never experienced such [a case] before. The child lived only three hours. (The notebook states that the child was a boy.)

1485. 1708 on 19 July fetched beyond Weerdeburen-over-Ee to Janke, wife of a labourer, after she had been three days in labour with a midwife. Found her desperate and feverish. Drank big beer glasses full [of] beer continuously, for which I scolded the midwife, who answered me, she wanted to have it. I said that the bladder would burst when the child was born. She answered me, she had drunk up a "rinckelmantie"[35] [of] beer in a quarter of an hour.[36] One could not look upon the body without fright. I did everything that art allowed. I gave her up so that she could be delivered by a man-midwife. The child was dead. But there was no man-midwife; he had gone to Bolsward. I had brought my instruments[37] with me already thinking that something must be wrong, because it was so far from my house. Then I said, [I] could help her, but if she came to die, they would slander me. But the woman in childbed insisted very much; I should still help her, so I was talked into it. I thrust my hook in the child's mouth; pulled it towards me. Immediately the bladder burst, so that the water ran over my whole body with such a noise as if a musket had been fired. But I helped the woman quickly with the instrument. And was fine. On the third day she demanded the [piss]pot. And the bladder was reduced again to her great fortune. She was delivered on [the] Monday evening; the Sunday after within a week she came two hours going to Dokkum. That was a miracle. I stayed with her, so [...?]. (The notebook claims that the other midwife had been with the woman two days, not three.)

1533. 1708 on 15 November fetched to Oostrum to Tetzke, wife of Chlas Elses, labourer. Found that the child came with its back before the birth canal. Was impossible to turn it, unless I put her bending forward with the head down. With great difficulty got the feet, brought them to the birth canal, put her again in her proper position. Got it with very great labour and difficulty, but then the birth canal closed around its head, which was malformed. And I had terrible work with it. But when it was born it was a big creature and dead. It was a pig's head, no nose, no bones behind. Very miserable, the hand three fingers with one nail, the other hand the fingers grown into each other, also one nail. The feet monstrous, to [the] great horror of us all. Oh Lord, save us from such cases. The people accused the woman of having worked so much around a young pig or farrow[38] when she was pregnant, that the creature must [have] always been with her, sitting with her at the table or on her lap. People may certainly take warning from this case, and not have such foolish ways.[39] (The notebook adds that the child was a boy. It had no bones at the back of its head and no palate.)

1609. 1709 fetched on 9 June to a dishonoured sweetheart called Brörrke, who was the daughter of the porter of The Three Pipes, Frerick. Delivered it with the feet. Very heavy. The water was already gone days before. It was very misformed in [its] hands and feet with short arms, first fat, then very thin. The feet also the same. Two fingers. A strange creature. It died in three weeks. The Lord punished her because she had sworn to herself that she should not get with child, that she knew better. It [the child] was from a doctor where she lived. (The notebook mentions that it was a boy.)

1626. 1709 on 1 August fetched to Gem[ke], wife of Frerick, cooper. Delivered her of two children: the first came right; I turned the other [and] delivered it with its feet. Helped her quickly. The string was between the legs [of] the child, so that it was held back. And had to cut it with razor in pieces. Then went quickly forward. The woman was very faint; she had to vomit continuously and she was very sick [throughout] the whole delivery. However, after the delivery healthy. The children lived one week. (The dairy adds that she delivered a son and a daughter. The second child came awkwardly.)

1656. 1709 on 23 November to Driesum to the wife of Hessel, carpenter; had been two midwives there. Had broken the water too early. Came with the hands first. Little or no opening. I had to make room. Turned it, delivered it by the feet with terrible difficulty because there was no opening there. A dead child. The mother does well. (The notebook extract mentions that the child's head got stuck fast.)

1671. 1710 on 25 January was fetched to Ecke, wife of Willem, copper repairer. Found that the child lay very high. Little labour. The vagina outside the body, which [had] been like this for half a year. Good council was hard to come by. I fomented her with "mother herbs" to soften it, but would not soften. Induced the labour, and the child must pass as if through a bowel. And another woman had to hold her vagina with both hands; the child must [pass] through there. Without that her whole womb and bowels and intestines would have followed [come out].[40] Days before she had got such shivering and cold, so that the child must then have been dead inside her. After the delivery I have laid her on her back and brought it inside the body. She was first well. But on the third day changed. Then the ninth day quiet. People said that she had taken very heavy drink from a quack doctor, who assured her, that she carried no child, but had a "suger" or a "vlyger".[41] That had been very strong physic as if she was a horse. Through this the woman became very unlucky. She was ailing in her pregnancy, which happens more often. (The notebook extract explains that after the delivery, while there was still an opening, Schrader got the womb and vagina back inside the body.)

1672. 1710 on 5 February with Jan Gorrtzacke's daughter, Hinke, whose husband, Wattse, was a corn merchant, who was visiting her mother. And delivered her quickly of a son. Lived but half an hour.

But, The Lord works mysteriously, I [was] terrified. Found that between the stomach and the belly [there] was an opening as big as a gold guilder, all round it grew a horny border. Out of this hung the intestines with the bowels. Had grown outside the body. One saw there the heart, liver, lungs clear and sharp, without decay. One could touch wholely under the breast. It was worthy to be seen by an artist, but she did not want it to be shown. I inquired [of] the woman if she had also had a fright or mishap. She declared that she was unaware of anything, but that [when] it had been the killing time they had slaughtered a pig. They had hung it on the meat hook, and the butcher had cut out the intestines and the bowels.

1728. 1710 fetched to Ternaard to Trijntie, wife of Jan Jansen, verger. A son. Delivered her after there had been a midwife from Ternaard with her two days. The child lay behind the pubic bone [ijsbeen]. Was stuck very fast. And it went very heavily. But through The Lord's help, helped her quickly.

1734. 1710 on 27 September fetched to Antie, wife of the brewer, Aate Schoyeles. By The Lord's decree, delivered her two daughters. The first came forth sitting. Broke the water of the other. He presented with his [...?]. I had to look for the feet. Got them with great difficulty, though delivered it with its feet. Still all well, by God's blessing, for mother and children. (The dairy states that the first child came with its bottom first, the second back first.)

1743. 1710 been fetched on 18 October to Hantum to the wife of Pitter Bockes, who had been in heavy labour for two whole days. And assisted by the midwife from Hantum and surgeon Nicklas, who both gave it over [to Schrader]. I found the arms born to the shoulder. Placed her backwards and not without great difficulty brought the shoulder and arm inside. Looked for the feet. The child was dead when I came. I had heavy work before I could get the feet. But The Lord be thanked. It progressed quickly. And the mother does well. (The notebook adds that the nape of the neck was also against the birth canal. Schrader delivered the child in a quarter of an hour.)

1795. 1711 on 10 February I was fetched to Nijkerk to Wattse Jennema, whose wife was called Alltie Jouwkes. She wanted me to attend her, but didn't call for me. And fetched a midwife from Morra, who tortured her for three days. She turned it over to the man-midwife, doctor Van den Berrg. He said, he must cut off the child's arms and legs. He took her for dead. And he said, the child was already dead. Then I was fetched in secret. When I came there her husband and friends were weeping a great deal. I examined the case, suspected that I had a chance to deliver [her]. The woman was very worn out. I laid her in a warm bed, gave her a cup of caudle[42], also gave her something in it; sent the neighbours home, so that they would let her rest a bit. An hour after her strength awakened again somewhat. And I had the neighbours fetched again. And after I had positioned the woman in labour, [I] heard that the doctor came then to sit by my side. I pulled the child to the birth canal and in half of a quarter of an hour I got a living daughter. And I said to the doctor, here is your dead child, to his shame. He expected to earn a hundred guilders there.[43] The friends and neighbours were very surprised. The mother and the child were in a very good state. (The notebook maintains that altogether it took Schrader three hours to deliver the child.)

1810. 1711 on 20 March fetched to Mayke, wife of Cornelis Jans, Mennonite preacher and thread winder. I was with her three days and nights doing everything which art allowed. The child came presented right, but was grown in fast. Have drawn off her water through a catheter; also given an enema. And everything in the presence of doctor Eysma. It was caused by all that heavy bearing down and the presentation of an arm. That was not good. The child was then already dead. I had to cut off an arm, and delivered it with terrible difficulty. And stuck the hook in the back of his head and got it like this. The Lord be praised, honoured and thanked. The woman does well. A healthy childbed. It is a woman who had always been very crippled in her lower body. Such [women] have heavy births and deliveries in general.[44] (The notebook adds that the woman retained her water. After the delivery the arm Schrader cut off was put in her sleeve, because she did not want anyone to see it. The woman was healthy and unharmed after the birth. The child was a boy.)

1824. 1711 on 28 April to Mayke, the wife of master Watse, a boat builder. The child came [presented] with his back sideways. She had a heavy flooding. With very great difficulty I pulled the child with its bottom to the birth canal. It was hard for her and myself. And had almost given it up, but The Lord gave deliverance. And had to be born doubled up with his bottom [presenting]. However the child and the mother lived. A healthy childbed.

1831. 1711 on 16 July (11 June) fetched to Wetzens to the wife of Chlas Jans, where Teyrtie the midwife had been. And she had delivered the child. I was fetched and examined her. Found that the rectum [was] very strained, the uterus black and inflamed. And got out several pieces of the afterbirth with my hand. The woman was in

death-like distress, and as if she had labour pains. When I had
delivered her of the afterbirth, [I] put my hand inside, brought the
womb to its place and helped the woman on with tincture of French
wine, [with] myrrh and alum added to it. And also a cataplasm.[45]
And then the pain stopped immediately. The woman healthy and
well recovered. (The notebook mentions that the husband was a
labourer. Schrader also found the neck of the womb in front of the
uterus when she came to the woman.)

1847. 1711 on 3 August I was fetched to Driesum to the wife of Gerrt Pyrs,
tailor. There had already been another midwife with her for one
whole day. I found the hands and the feet together in the birth
canal. The navel string outside the birth canal. The child was dead. I
pulled the head to [the] side, looked for the feet and helped her in a
quarter of an hour to [the] great gladness and wonder of the
bystanders. The child had got a rupture of its navel [while it was] in
the mother's body as big as [...?]. (The notebook informs us that the
rupture was as big as a duck's egg. The woman was doing well.)

1880. 1711 on 14 October I was fetched to Ternaard to Antie, the wife of
Chlas, carrot buyer. Found that the water was already gone the day
before. Little opening. A hard lopsided womb. Lay with his
shoulders in front of the birth canal; had one hand forward. I had to
lay her face forwards. Got it from behind. I turned the feet to the
birth canal. Placed her again in position and got it with great
difficulty. Then stayed motionless. The womb shut round his neck.
Then had to put a string around the child's neck, and delivered it
with great force. Had I been then before the water was broken and
the midwife from Ternaard had been there, I could have helped her
better and helped her easily. The woman had a healthy childbed.
(The notebook extract adds that the woman was saved, but the
child dead. The other midwife, Detie Moy, had given the case up.)

1888. 1711 on 1 November fetched to Oosterwolde to Antie, the wife of a
man called Forrmer Jans, after the midwife had tormented her
there for two days. The [navel] string [was] outside the body, a sign
of the child's death. It was stuck in the side and with the head
crooked behind the pubic bone [ijsbeen]. Put her on her back, the
feet and the body high. Then got it in this way. [It was] hard. A dead
son. The woman does well. Oh Lord, You be thanked. (The
notebook extract states that the other midwife had only been there
one whole day.)

1943. 1712 on 11 March I was fetched to the toll-house at Driesum to
Locke, wife of a cattle dealer, after the midwife from Westergeest
had already been with her for two days. I found that the child lay

with his head between his legs. The child was already dead. Also it could never have been born in this manner [position]. Laid her bending over, head first in a woman's lap. And saved it in this way from behind. Put the woman in position again. Delivered [it] by the feet. That went quickly. The woman does well. (Again the notebook extract claims that the other midwife, Trintie Moy, had been there only for one whole day. The notebook account also claims that the child got stuck by its head for a long time when Schrader was delivering it. It was a boy.)

1975. 1712 on 4 August in The Kuikhaan to Simon, a labourer [the woman in childbirth] being the sister of Jackopes Backer from Dokkum, who persuaded me to travel so far.[46] [When I] came there, I found no people but her husband standing before the door. The labouring woman on a wet bundle of straw. And was stiff with cold. Water and flooding, it had all flowed out of her. She lay unconscious. I was angry with the man, saying how could people live so with a woman vomiting to her death. He said two midwives, also a man-midwife, had already been there with her, who had all left her with the women of the neighbourhood. I said he should immediately call the women of the neighbourhood again, which came to pass [and] I scolded those people [who] would give [someone] up to a miserable death without assistance or pity. Immediately the people got fire from the neighbours and I threw away the wet straw and made her a place to lie, put her a cap on. She lay stark naked. I positioned her, and took her for dead. And then examined how it was with the case. Found that the child lay with its stomach before the birth canal. It was rotten. A stinking flood. I turned it and delivered it in half of a quarter of an hour. The woman got so much strength again, sat up and wanted to kiss my hand. I comforted her, helped her to bed, where I revived her with some drops of warm beer, because there was nothing else to give. Three hours after that she died. The people told me, that she was tortured for two days by the midwives and the man-midwife. Oh such miserable know nothings, who mistreat their fellow-men in this way. (The notebook adds that the child was delivered by the feet.)

1984. 1712 on 24 August I was fetched to Akkerwoude to Meyndert Jans, who was nicknamed dirty Affke Moy. Her daughter had been in labour two days. Also had had two other midwives, who gave her over. I had to make a bad case from a good straightforward one. The child was dead when I came. But had to turn it with great difficulty, and delivered it by the feet. It was heavy [work]. The mother was in a good state. (The notebook mentions that Schrader had to put the woman face downward in order to deliver her.)

1993. 1712 on 7 September fetched to Driesum to a farmer called Ubele. Found that the child came with its knees first. It was impossible to get it straight by the feet. Had to lay her twice face downward with her head in a woman's lap. Got it with great difficulty by the feet. (The notebook entry claims that the child came with both its knees and face first. Schrader had much to do to deliver the woman. The child was dead, dying during the labour.)

2047. 1722 on 3 February was fetched to Oostersingel to Frans Fopes's daughter, whose husband was a skipper, where the midwife, Pittie Moy, had long procrastinated. I was fetched there [and] asked her how the case was proceeding. The child, she said, came with his genitals before the birth canal; it is a boy. I examined the case. But, oh heavens, how horrified I was. The child had no head. In place of that a swelling like a flat turnip, with sharp bones like thorns set around it. One could not touch without injuring the hands. I said, I could not help her; she had to be helped with an instrument. Surgeon Frans Berrger was fetched. When he examined her [he] said, I have delivered so many children, but never a headless child. And also had terribly much to do there before he could deliver her. The woman was well afterwards. (The notebook adds that the other midwife could not help her through "hand art". The child was rotten. Lord save us from such creatures.)

2075. 1723 on 21 May was fetched to Lisbit, the wife of Eelke Henderickx, who was a currier. The woman had a fairly easy labour, but, oh horror, the child had a fantastic growth on his head. And full curls all grown like meat. I asked her if she had ever mused about such things. She said, that she didn't know, but that she had always had a liking for children with curls like this on their forehead beneath a hat. If she had [a] child, she would also want that. But the child only lived an hour luckily for her. How careful the pregnant woman must be to conduct herself well in all she says and thinks.

2090. 1724 on 27 January fetched to Ipkie, wife of Jackop Isacks, confectioner. Delivered of two sons. The first came well [position-ed], the last came with [its] hands and feet like a round ball. Had to disentangle it. It lay very strangely. Delivered it with the feet, but everything well for the mother and children.

2114. 1724 on 20 September outside the Hanspoort to Titzke, wife of Tiese, butcher. Found that the water was broken without labour. Took until [the] evening at eight o'clock. Delivered her of a son, but the afterbirth stayed stuck over the whole womb. I didn't know where I should begin. I took her for dead. And I was busy with her for a good half hour. Had to pluck it off as people do with feathers from a duck. And fifty or more bits and pieces [were] plucked off, which made me almost faint from the effort. I had almost given her up, but everything through The Lord's help turned out well to my great astonishment. And the woman is healthy and well in her childbed and continues healthy. The previous year she had also been like this, and then had to call doctor Winnter from Leeuwarden, who delivered her. And the remainder [of the afterbirth] was driven away with potions. Oh Lord, save me in future from such encounters. (The notebook adds that she was fetched on Wednesday morning. She delivered the child without labour. Here Schrader claims that she pulled off a good 25 pieces of afterbirth.)

2116.   1724 on 13 November I was fetched to Hycke, wife of Alle Sickes, after the [another] midwife had been fetched there in the afternoon. She assured the woman, that she would be delivered at seven o'clock, and that it was a good, straightforward case. But she made a mistake. She thought that she had the head first [presenting], but it was the buttocks. A foot also came out of the birth canal. She laboured incessantly, to bring it in, thinking that it was a hand. And [did] that a good thirty times. She should have fetched the foot towards her and she should have looked for the other as well and have delivered [the child]. When I came the leg hung outside and was black. The child dead. I looked for the other foot and delivered it. The mother [is] saved. Oh [what a] wretch, such [a] messy bungler, who so mistreated [her] fellow-men. (The notebook gives the occupation of Alle Sickes as a girdle maker. It also names the other midwife as Pittie Moy.)

2119.   1724 on 8 December I was informed that there [was] a merchant's wife, whose name was Gerit Creemer, whose wife, Hilltie, had a heavy flooding for 14 days and nights. She was worn out. She sought my advice. I said to her, that her midwife must deliver her immediately. She asked me if I was troubled in my mind about being able to deliver a woman without labour. I said, in such instances, yes. The midwife had been with her for three days. Finally on one evening everyone thought that she must die. Then they came to fetch me late in the evening with a horse sledge. I was unwilling to go, but if the woman would have died, my conscience would have much troubled me. So I resolved [to go], still with resentment. Went along. When I came there I found the woman unconscious. Everyone thought that she was dead. I positioned her in order to examine her. I had some spirits, put them under the nose and [on] the pulses, and then I examined the case. Then she opened her eyes and feeling came back. I found that the afterbirth lay before the entrance of the child and delivered her of it. And looked for the child's feet and delivered it. But it was dead. And the skin was falling off. And then I let the woman rest still. I gave her a little something and [in the] morning [she] was completely another person. And the woman continued to improve later. If I had not saved the case, she surely would not have lived long. (The notebook adds that the case was in Ternaard. Schrader had to make an opening in order to deliver the woman. The notebook entry claims that the woman was delivered of a living child. The mother and child continued to improve.)

2132. 1725 on 1 March I was fetched to the Hanspoort to Ytie, wife of Balling, miller. The afterbirth lay before the entrance and [was] grown in fast. She had had heavy flooding for 14 days. Was no opening; had to make one. Looked for the feet with great difficulty. And had to fetch the afterbirth out in many pieces. Had almost given up, but The Lord strengthened me and brought solution. The child was smothered by the flooding. The mother [had] a healthy childbed. (The notebook extract mentions that Schrader took the afterbirth out in a good fifty pieces. Was a very heavy birth. The woman improved after the birth, but the child was dead.)

2137. 1725 on Easter morning (2 April) to Gertruyt, wife of master Heere, tailor, where the midwife Pytye Moy had been the whole night, but could not make progress. I also had heavy work there, because the face had to be avoided. But after heavy labour the mother [was] saved. But the child's face was swollen and puffy, but in the following days got somewhat better. (The notebook entry clarifies the fact that the child was born with its face presenting. Its face was hurt.)

2183. 1726 on 4 January been to Rinsumageest to Acke, wife of Rittsert, who was a dairyman. Had very heavy labour for two days. The child came with its face first, the birth canal closed around its neck. Therefore must be choked. And finally had to deliver it with the hook or instrument. The woman does well. (The notebook extract mentions that the child was stuck for two hours in the birth canal. The child was a boy.)

2185. 1726 on 14 March to my daughter, Schrader. Found that the child came very high. Then with his face before the birth canal. There was an expanded water, which I broke. Then turned the child quickly and delivered it by its feet. And otherwise a heavy birth for the mother and the child would have followed. Everyone thought that the child was dead, but revived again. A good son, Ernest Willem. Mother and child are in a good state.

2192. 1726 on 20 April [fetched] to Catelijn, the wife of Johanes Hollkes, town councillor, who was the daughter of the Mayor Lindeman. Fourteen days before she got very bad pains in her leg and bad intermittent fits, the intermittent fits lasting for three days, but [got] better again. I had great difficulty. Had to foment her over a warm bath. Was no opening. Had to make it myself. But in the end everything well for mother and child. (The notebook extract gives the date of this case as Sunday, 28 April. Also it states that the woman was delivered of a dead, rotten daughter.)

2205. 1726 on 3 August outside the Aalsumerpoort to Antie, wife of Reynerr, smith. I delivered her two sons. The first came well, but the second could not break the water sack into pieces. Had to break it with [something] sharp.[47] Turned the child with great difficulty. It lay very awkwardly with the shoulder before the birth canal. But delivered it still living. The afterbirth was also grown in. Very difficult, but everything still well for mother [and] children. (The notebook adds that the second child could not break the water sack because it was so thick. Schrader got the second child by its feet, with the heels upwards. Were very big, heavy children. The deliveries were accompanied by much flooding.)

2240. 1727 on 3 January to Ynsske, wife of Volkert Bouwes, potter. Found that the water was gone. The opening like a "beesem-stuivertie"[48]. I had to make room with my hands, but was difficult because of [a] hard womb. In the end I got hold of the feet. And had no room above [for] half a "schellinck".[49] However, fetched it with great force towards me. If God was not almighty, it could never have been born: also the child was very monstrous. The head was so very thick and full of water[50], that I had to make an opening in it, so the water flowed out of it. The body also heavy with water. Punctured it through with my fingers and so The Lord still gave it me. I can never forget the miracles concerning The Lord's great deeds. The child had no nose or mouth, no roof of the mouth; otherwise it was in order. The Lord save me further from such happenings. The woman [was] first rosy and healthy. The Lord be believed and praised. (The notebook adds that Schrader attended the case on Friday evening. The woman was a currier's daughter. She continued to do well.)

2261. 1727 on 13 April, the second Easter Day with Zitke Mijns, wife of Caarel, dairyman. Found the water gone. The child with its back before the birth canal. Had to turn it. Went very heavily. Little room. I had almost given it up, but The Lord gave me strength and once more gave blessing, so that fortunately mother and child were saved. (The notebook states that the child was a girl. Schrader delivered her by the feet.)

2265. 1727 on (Saturday) 3 May was fetched to Trintie, the wife of the Mayor Synya. The water was already gone. The naval string outside. The child dead. And lying on [its] side. Must be choked, because the string hung outside. I had much trouble and work before I could get hold of the feet. But The Lord gave [the child] quickly. I saved it. The woman does well. (The dairy extract says that it was necessary to choke the child because Schrader could not deliver it without using great force. A dead daughter.)

2292. 1727 on (Monday) 8 September with Mayke, wife of Gerrit Jans, a a long distance skipper. I delivered her immediately of three children. The first came with its back forward [presenting]. Turned it, delivered it quickly with the feet. The second came right a quarter of an hour after the first. Was a girl. The third came more awkwardly. Turned it, delivered it immediately. Was also already rotting. This was a boy. Only the middle one stayed alive. I believed the reason for the death [of] these two children [was] because the mother had [lain] three or four weeks in [a] heavy fever [and] had suffered very death-like oppressiveness. But a fortunate delivery and moreover a healthy childbed [for the mother]. (The notebook gives a somewhat different account of the case. Schrader claims that the third child was a girl. The second child, which lived, was a boy. The first child was also already rotten.)

2313. 1728 on 14 January with Gebke, wife of Laas, turf cutter, after I had suffered heavy labour with the woman there, and had examined everything [for] four to five hours. Could not make progress. In such circumstances one can and must pay attention as to whether there is something amiss which obstructs the delivery. I brought my hand inside; the child lay very squashed like a round ball. I disentangled it. And [it] would have been impossible [for it] to be born like this. And [I] had to make a bad birth from a good one; delivered it undamaged by the feet. I had not thought that such [a] desirable outcome was possible. It was like a miracle. And the mother and child are fresh and healthy. (The notebook entry adds that the child was a boy and that Schrader was with her during about three hours of heavy labour.)

2347. 1728 on 23 [November] with Jelltie, wife of Jan Minnes, baker. And found Rymke, the midwife, with her. And I had to [...?] Rymke. The woman in labour did not want to be tortured any longer by her. I examined the case; found that she was very closed tight. I said, one must show some patience. I wanted to go back home, but the husband, wife and friends didn't want to be without me. I took the work in The Lord's name and saved the mother and child. The woman delivered patiently and quietly, while before I came she moaned and shrieked terribly. I helped her within an hour. Everything still well for mother and child. The Lord's name be thanked. (The notebook adds that Schrader took over the case from Rymke. The child remained a long time in the birth canal. It was a girl, who died in 13 days without pain or suffering.)

2404. The year 1729 on 26 August [called to] Une, a toll keeper, [who was] nicknamed Ramsnoes[51]. I was called to her, after Trintie, her mother, who was also a midwife from Rinsumageest, had tortured her daughter for two days. She give it up. And had made bad work. Came with its bottom before the birth canal. A stiff womb. I got the feet, but with great effort. The child and the mother were well. But the child died the same day.

2421. 1726 [1729] on 26 November with Pyttie, wife of Tys Wouwter de Haan, geneva[52] distiller and town councillor. Found that she was in great pain. The water broke. The child still did not present itself. Lay high behind the pubic bone [ijsbeen] with his back [presenting]. A very heavy birth. Tried to turn it, but even with great trouble almost could not get it. The second foot was still worse. Had to bend her [the woman in labour] forward with her head down. Got [it] with terrible difficulty. Then still stayed with the head stuck fast, but still got it. The child lived, but not long. The mother was well. (The notebook adds that the child was a girl.)

2431. 1729 on 18 December with Liwkie, wife of Jan Henderickx, master shoemaker. Lingered long. I found that it [came] with its bottom before the birth canal. I tried to place it before the birth canal, but in vain. I looked for the feet; could only do it using great force. I had terribly much difficulty to do this because the child was monstrous and watery, head and chest. A very frightful head. It had no mouth or roof of the mouth. Oh Lord, save us from such creatures. It was dead. The mother [had] a healthy childbed. (The dairy extract states that the delivery took place on Sunday morning. The mother was well following the birth. A son.)

2441. 1730 on 10 February (Thursday night) fetched to Antie, wife of Wybe Chlassen, peddler. Found that [the] head, hands and feet lay in a round ball in front of the birth canal. With terrible difficulty [I] had to place the child upward and look for the feet. The people who were there and I were very astonished that the child could have stayed alive and undamaged. It proceeded with great difficulty. And mother and child are well. God's works are great.

2465. 1730 on 30 May fetched to Siwkie, wife of Luttyen, cooper. Found that she had a lopsided womb. I had to make all the openings and arrange the womb on one side. It took a long time. And stayed motionless. Then I thought, there has to be something wrong. Did an examination; the child sat with arms and legs behind the pubic bone [ijsbeen] and with his face upwards. A dangerous birth. Had to lie her [the woman in labour] face downward. Turned it twice. Very heavy. And delivered it with the feet. The mother and the child are well; The Lord be thanked. It was an extraordinary case. Had almost given it up, but The Lord strengthened me with more than usual power. Oh praise [be]. (The notebook entry adds that the delivery took from four o'clock in the morning till the afternoon. Schrader had to put the mother on her head twice. Got the child with its feet from behind. Delivered it using great force. Schrader had not thought that the child could still be alive and undamaged. She thanks The Lord who had saved her from danger a thousand times. And once again her sighs and prayers were heard and He rejoiced in her victory, so that mother and child were healthy and safe. A daughter.)

2469. 1730 on 11 June fetched to Catharina, wife of Jan Teyrckx, baker. Took from Saturday night to Sunday evening. The labour was all over. And I went away, but [in the] evening it [the labour] came back again, after the water was already gone the day before. The child stayed for a good hour in the birth canal and could not deliver [it]. But then I let her stand and got it standing. A daughter. Came right. I found that there was still another [child], but that lay very entangled between the afterbirth, with a very strong water sack. Could almost not break it. The child came with the back forward [presenting]. Looked for the feet; got it like this. All well for mother and children. The children both died the next day. (The notebook states that the delivery took till Sunday evening at seven o'clock. The labour stopped for six hours, although the child was in the birth canal. At the end of the afternoon labour began again. The second child was a boy. Both died five or six hours after the birth. The mother remained well.)

2520. 1731 on 27 February with Anna, wife of master Kurt Sirrks, master shoemaker. Found a lopsided womb. And had to make the opening with my hands and fingers to the end. It was very heavy work. And pulled the child out [of] her with force and strength. And managed then. Still well for the mother and child. A son.

2569. 1731 on (Tuesday), 1 August with Jetzke, wife of Jan, servant of geneva distiller, Jackop Jetses. Had lived together twenty years, without ever having had a child. Came three months after her time. She could not be helped without "hand art". The child stuck fast with his head. Had very much to do with it [the delivery]. She was old in years. Had to press the head very flat before it could be born through such a narrow passage. But after the birth, I got the head right again. The mother and child well. (The notebook states that the child was a boy.)

2571. 1731 on 8 August fetched to Siwkie, wife of Berrent Ellties, butcher. Found a heavy lopsided womb. A very big fat child. Could almost not be born. Stayed with the shoulders stuck fast. I worked almost above my strength. At last The Lord gave relief. And mother and child were well. (The notebook adds that the woman delivered a son.)

2594. 1731 on Friday, 13 October been fetched to Bauwkie, wife of Jan Lambers, who was a bargeman. And I was busy with her till Monday. Put all means, internally and externally, to work, but could not progress further. At last [the] people decided to call a man-midwife, Frans Berrger, who [used] very much work and force. He said the arm or elbow lay behind [the] pubic bone [ijsbeen]. Had to first break the arm and open the head. Using all force, could almost not get hold of it. It was stuck. But at last delivered of a big, dead daughter. The woman was stable at first. A day after she got a bad pain in the body and the looseness. Died [on] the twelfth day. (The notebook mentions that Schrader was called to the case in the evening. Was busy with the case till Monday morning. The delivery lasted for three whole days. Had to extract the child with a hook. The notebook claims that the woman was well after the delivery, and does not mention her death.)

2596. 1731 on 18 October with Rickst, wife of Pitter Derckx, seaman. Found that there [was] a lopsided womb and fast closed womb. I foresaw a heavy delivery. To the end I had to make all the room with my fingers. And it was very hard. And I had terribly heavy work there to the end. A big, heavy child. The Lord be thanked. Mother and child are both well. (The notebook extract adds that the delivery took one whole day. A fine daughter.)

2598. 1731 on (Tuesday) 22 October fetched in the night to Hantum to Pitternelletie Wirrsma, wife of minister Brugman. And the water was already gone when I came. A miraculous delivery. I had much to do. The child could almost not be born; it was so entangled. [The naval string] four times around its neck, back and arms. But succeeded. Heavy son. (The notebook adds that the woman was delivered between noon and one o'clock [on Wednesday].)

2626. 1732 on 6 March with Grittie Minnes, wife of Cornelis Jans, innkeeper. Found that the water was already gone. Sat with its private parts before the birth canal. And was very perilous [work] to save the child. But with very cautious help it [came] at last out of the birth canal. Placed it with its buttocks forward [presenting]. Got it doubled up. I broke a second water and delivered a second child. Two good sons. All well. (The notebook adds that the first child's sack stayed for a long time in the birth canal. The second child came right and quickly into the birth canal.)

2640. 1732 on 12 April (Easter night) fetched to Trintie, wife of Ducke Jans, master ship's carpenter. Found that a very heavy labour [was] on hand. A lopsided womb, the face upwards and no opening. It was terrible. And I worked above my strength. And we both had it very heavy. Finally, The Lord gave deliverance. All still well for mother and child. (The notebook states that the delivery took until evening the following day, 13 April.)

2653. 1732 on 28 [=26 v.L.] May fetched outside the Hanspoort to Coy, wife of Wopke, [ship's] carpenter. Found that the child [lay] sideways in front of the birth canal with one buttock before the birth canal. She and I had it very heavy. The child had a heavy head. [The head] would almost not follow, but finally all well for mother and child. (The notebook mentions that the delivery took place on Monday evening. Schrader delivered the child, a son, by its feet.)

2668. 1732 on 28 July with Mayke, wife of Pouwelus Scheltes. Had little opening and also little labour. Had to help everything along through art. Lasted from Monday evening till Tuesday. And it was a very heavy and difficult birth. It was stuck fast in the closed up womb. And had to make it loose from the inside. A small child. Found that there was still one more. That came with both its hands first. Turned it, delivered it by the feet, but a dead fruit [child]. But all well for the woman. Oh Lord, save me in the future. (The notebook adds that the husband was a labourer. The case took until Tuesday afternoon. Schrader almost gave up, but with The Lord's help at last got the first child, which finally presented right. The second child presented with both its hands and head. Both the children were boys.)

2686. 1732 on 16 September with Lisbeit Hogacker, wife of Keesie, the son of Jackop Sybeltie. Got a daughter. And the child had on its back a circle like the palm of a hand with [a] callus; there was a wall around with an opening to the inside, there was a membrane grown over, containing bloody water.[53] But died on the third day. The Lord will save us from things like this. (The notebook gives the occupation of the husband as a shoemaker.)

2771. 1733 on 10 November with Maryken, wife of the servant to the orphanage. A son. But had a face like an ape. At the back of the neck an opening as big as a hand. Its genitals were also not as they should be. She [the mother] had seen apes dancing. It did not live long. Oh Lord, save us from such monsters.

2809. 1734 on 21 April with Anderis, butcher on the Streek, [to] Catharina, daughter of Hinne Faaber. Found a lopsided womb. The child in the side, squeezed very tightly. And had a heavy labour before I got it loose. And I had to work above my nature [strength]. A very terrible labour. But everything still fortunate for mother and child. Oh Lord, praise and thanks.[54]

2817. 1734 with Geesken, wife of Johans Rinckx, merchant-skipper [and] delivered two sons. Both lay very awkwardly. Had to turn both to [get] the feet. The last sat very high up. Could not get hold of one foot without great difficulty. But managed. Quickly. All well.

2818. 1734 on 8 August outside the Hanspoort [to the] labourer to the tile works, the daughter of Reyner Sup, farmer. Was no opening. Came with its face upwards. Stayed with its head stuck fast. Got it with its feet. Got it loose with terrible work. The bystanders and I thought [that] the child must be dead. But, The Lord be thanked, to all our astonishment it lived. Everything well for mother and child.

2819. 1734 on 9 August with Antie, daughter of Teyrt Ipes, wife of Gerrt Minnes, miller. And found the child with its back before [...?]. Had to save it. Placed her [the woman in labour] face downward on her head. Looked for the feet, which lay very high in the body. Got them with much difficulty. Still everything well for mother and child.

2820. 1734 with Jette, wife of Chlas Janssen, shoemaker and tradesman, after she had fallen from the attic and [was] dreadfully hurt underneath her body, with a very heavy flooding. Was still twelve weeks to go and then delivered of a well-formed daughter. And then everything was still well to [my] great surprise. God's works are great.

2821. 1734 on 6 September with Antie, wife of Zirrick Ydes, sailor to Greenland. Had a very heavy delivery, because the child had a very heavy head and broad shoulders. Could almost not be born. The Lord gave me more than ordinary strength, so that I managed through God's miracles. All well for mother and child.

2822. This is an remarkable, curious case. 1734 on 20 November I was fetched at twelve o'clock at night to Siwke, wife of Berent Ellties, butcher. And her labour had come in the late afternoon, but she dared not fetch me, because they were slaughtering and the house was full of men folk. It was not the right thing to do. [They] could have brought me with her to another room. When I came at night there was nothing to do. And there were signs, that there would soon be a delivery. She drank tea with saffron. Then laid her next to her husband on the bed, and she insisted that I went home, because there was nothing to be done. But I wanted to stay with her, thinking it would change in the bed in the warmth. And we sat with the three or four of us talking; knowing no anxiety, she slept well. An hour after she got, waking up, such [a] terrible cold fever, that I had never heard of [before] in my life. That lasted half an hour. We took her from the bed to a big fire. Fomented her under and above. Finally she got such a great temperature, she could not endure it. I said, we must walk. Then I said, we must make the bed again and lie you then again in a warm bed. Then you must go home [the woman said]. No, I said, we shall first see what this strange fever will bring us. And before you go to bed, I shall first look if a change has resulted from this. So she said, I shall first make water. She got the pot and was alright. She gave a snort and fell from the pot, and was soon completely dead. Together with the husband we were all dead shocked. We then brought her to a stool. While we were bringing her there the child came. It lay under her without [her being in] labour; that was [probably] caused by the fever. The child lived; has reached two years of age. Oh curious case.

2823. 1735 on 3 February with Rickxst, wife of Jan Aarens, basket maker. Found that the child lay on its side with the mouth before the birth canal, and as if the neck would break. [I] had terrible difficulty to bring it to rights. Was impossible [for] me. Had to manipulate everything. And it was a very heavy labour. The Lord worked still miraculously through me, through his all-powerful strength and goodness, so that mother and child are well.

2906. 1736 on (Sunday), 28 October with Trintie, wife of the son of Johanes Reynouws, labourer to the tile makers. Found an expanded water, which broke. It presented the right arm with the string in the birth canal. Brought them in again together. Looked with very great difficulty for the feet, that lay very high. Had to put her on her head. Could still not [get it]. Pulled for [such a] long [time] towards me, that at last got one foot away from behind the pubic bone [ijsbeen]. Then still remained with the womb closed around its neck. It was very dangerous for mother and child. The child was dead; the mother does well. (The notebook extract adds that the child also got stuck with its chin behind the pubic bone [ijsbeen]. It was a boy.)

2933. 1738 on (Sunday evening), 21 April fetched outside the Hanspoort
to Catharina Faber, the daughter of Anderis, butcher. A very heavy
labour. The child had a very malformed head. Was stuck in the side.
Took a full six hours or so. And I had terribly hard work. It came
out for the best for the mother. Had a healthy childbed. The child
lived three hours. It was very malformed; short arms, strange
hands, the legs also not right, no private parts. The Lord save all
people from such happenings. The woman had always such heavy
births. And before my time was already delivered once by a
surgeon, but I still have always helped her.

2956. 1739 on (Friday), 22 May with Haabeltie Vockeda, wife of
Henderick Teyrtz, merchant. Delivered her of two children. The
first and biggest was born dead. The second, very delicate, lived.
Turned them and delivered them with the feet. Quickly. All well.
(The notebook states that the first child was a boy, the second a girl.
The second child lived for nine days.)

2969. 1739 on (Saturday night), 29 September with Ninke Boeck, wife of
Waade Derckx, geneva distiller's labourer. A very heavy labour,
because she was very crippled on both sides. Also too small and
delicate. The child could only pass through the pubic bones, with
difficulty, because they were so closed up. And she and I had it very
heavy. But The Almighty God made everything still come out for
the best. A good son. And all well for mother and child. The Lord
be thanked.

2978. 1740 last February [on] Shrove Tuesday in the evening I have been
fetched to Betterwird to Titzke, wife of Binne Maarten, farmer. She
complained that [for] a full week she had had such a severe shaking
through all her limbs, with such trembling that people became
concerned. And that still lasted into labour. It [the delivery] did not
progress. [With] every labour pain the child went back up, till at last
it came [was born]. Then the child was so strangely entangled
together, round the arms and legs, back [and] neck, and was in a
round ball. After the delivery the trembling stopped. And have
never known anything similar. I think that this would have caused
this strange entanglement. The mother and the child are well. (The
notebook extract mentions that the child was a boy. Schrader was
paid five guilders by the mother. Ietke Moy gave 22 stuivers.)

2979. 1740 on 23 May been fetched to Pittie, wife of Cornelis X, school-
master. And found that she had heavy flooding. And already before
I came to her [was it] so, that all her life's strength was gone away.
And without the least labour. Administered a heart strengthener to
her, in order to stop the flooding. I stayed the whole night. In the

morning I let the minister be fetched, who said a prayer. Thereafter I resolved to deliver her without labour, in order to save her, if it was possible. I took her for dead; she had no more strength. The afterbirth was loose, which caused the distress and the heavy flooding. Now The Lord commanded the work of my hands, and I got a dead, rotten son. The Lord be thanked. The mother is saved and with time got her former strength again, to the wonder of us all. God's miracles are great. (The notebook entry adds that the case was in Aalsum.)

2980. Now I was one day after this above case again called to such a happening. 1740 on 24 May to Oostrum to Antie, wife of Ullbe Bewalde; where the minister Brantzma was there, and she lay in a dead faint. And [the] people said to me, that she had bled a [bean]bucketful of blood. The midwife had left her. I gave her a little something; the flooding abated. I stayed the whole night with her. The next day I went away again. Then were two days without flooding. Then it [the flooding] came so quickly over her again; they fetched me immediately. I looked if I could possibly get the child, but she struggled [the woman] with death. And [I] also took her for dead. All her strength and life's juices were gone. I still got the child with force. Could not get it from her because the child [was] dead and she [the mother] could not assist with it. She still saw the child. Then she shut her eyes and died, the good woman, to [the] great sadness of her husband, son and parents and us all. Oh Lord, save me further from such deliveries [as these] two. (The notebook extract adds that when the flooding stopped she was stable. This state lasted from Sunday till Tuesday. When the flooding started again the afterbirth was in the mouth of the womb. And it was grown in fast around the child's head. Turned the child, and delivered it with its feet. A very heavy fat son.)

The Lord knows whether this shall be my last [case]. I hope so. It will be so.

Now I have had more than a hundred bad and heavy complicated births. There was much writing involved. Of these mentioned all were dangerous. And yet there is not one of them, whether or not they had the life and bodily health left to them, that The Lord alone had not ordained; otherwise it would have been impossible many times. Him alone the praise. Not me, Oh Lord, but all praise should be Yours; laudation, praise, honour and glory till eternity. Only this last has died in childbirth, but she wrestled already with death when I came to her. I have seen over this, and to my wonder, [the memoirs

niu ben jck een daug na dit vor nomde qual wer bij
so ein so vul gehalt

1740 den 24 mej tot osterum bij ullbe bewalde
sijn vrouw antie dar de predikant krantz mu
bij war en sij in een dodelicke flauwte lag
en men seijde mij datse wel een koon emmer
bloet gesleijt hadde de vroet vrouw hade haar
verlaten ick ordenerde haar wat de vloet stilde
ick bleff de heele nacht bij haar ander dags
vertrock ick waer was don 2 daayen sonder
vloet don gwam het haar wer so hastig ouer
haalden mij an stontz ick ondersoyt of ick
het kint nit maytij konde worden mar sij
werrstelde met de doodt en nam haar ock
ver doodt an al haar chrayten en linens
soppen wauran wey ick knej het kint nog
met gewelt konde het nit van haar krijgen
om dat het kint doodt en sij gen sulp so brengen
konde sij heft het kint nog gesijn doen stoel
sij haar voyen en sterf so haar dij kraue
vrouw tot grutte drofhiet van haar man
soen en oiwaurs en ons alle o heer bewar
mij verder ver sulcke 2 vornellen

of dit nu ver mijn leste sal weesen, ij de Heer
Bekent ick hoop van jaa het sij soo

Page from the Notebook of Vrouw Schrader (folio 487)

are] there to be used as a guide, or after my death, so someone still may get use or learning from it, to the advantage of my fellow-men.

I have [written] this in my eighty-fifth year of old age, 1740 on 18 September. And it shall now be my last light. And I have during the time of my sinful life had a heavy time. And about over four thousand children helped into the world, these including 64 twins and three triplets.
Catharina G. Schraders, widow of Mayor Higt.

NOTES

1. The names of persons appearing in the cases have been transcribed as they appear in the original manuscript. Place names have been converted to their modern spelling. Where place names have ceased to exist, the most recent version has been given, taken mainly from Ch.H. van Aken, *Aardrijkskunding Woordenboek Der Geheele Aarde*, 4th edition, Rotterdam: Nijgh & van Ditmars Uitg., 1926.
2. In this and many other cases Schrader mentions the fact that she found it "necessary" to pull the afterbirth loose, often with force. During this period it was believed vital to extract the placenta immediately after birth, for fear that the cervix would close up and prevent its exclusion. Although some midwives apparently allowed it to be delivered naturally, it was often considered better practice and proof of greater skill if the midwife "fetched" it. In the late 17th century the Dutch obstetrician Van Deventer suggested that the best method was to sweep round the uterus with the hand to remove the placenta and debris. See Audrey Eccles, *Obstetrics and Gynaecology in Tudor and Stuart England*, 92.
3. Vrouw Schrader makes frequent reference in the notebook extracts to The Lord's help and mercy in guiding her through difficult deliveries. She also makes numerous pleas to be "saved in the future from such terrible births". Because these statements recur so frequently they have not, unless they are of particular significance, been taken up from the notebook entries.
4. In some of the cases information additional to, or differing from, that given in the memoirs appears in the notebook. The supplementary items in parenthesis denote additional information lifted from the notebook accounts.
5. Friesland, the region where Vrouw Schrader lived and worked, is the North-Western-most province of The Netherlands, a region subject to harsh winter weather conditions. Dissected as it is by rivers and lakes, the terrain presented severe problems of transportation for Schrader when travelling to deliveries. In this passage she mentions travelling by sleigh; in future extracts barges and sailing boats, sometimes to islands off Friesland.
6. The distance between Hallum and Wijns is only approximately eight kilometers, yet this was further than Schrader usually travelled to attend cases. The difficulties encountered during this journey further emphasise the problems of transportation faced by Vrouw Schrader.
7. Leeuwarden is the provincial capital of Friesland, approximately six kilometers from Wijns (and thirteen kilometers from Hallum).
8. The word "benauwd" translates literally as "oppressive". This may appear to be a

curious way of describing childbirth, but is peculiarly apt when we remember the fear of death which surrounded childbearing during this period.

9. Schrader makes frequent reference to her efforts to deliver women "by art" ("kunst") or using "hand art". This would seem to indicate a degree of intervention and manipulation, but also the application of skill, knowhow, expertise, handiness, dexterity, and artistry.

10. Schrader refers in her memoirs to three classes of medical practitioner apart from midwives "meesters" (surgeons), "doctors" (physicians) and "vroedmeysters" (man-midwives or accoucheurs).

11. Here Schrader makes reference to a constant and often justified fear amongst midwives, that of women dying under their hands during the delivery. When in doubt Schrader seems to have preferred to call in a surgeon or man-midwife, not necessarily to supervise or intervene, but to act as a witness to her actions in the case.

12. In many of the cases described in the memoirs several midwives from neighbouring villages and towns were called to the delivery scene. This was the usual practice in more complicated cases, a surgeon or man-midwife being summoned most often as a last resort. The presence of a man in the delivery room signalled the use of instruments to complete the birth, and all too frequently the abandonment of hope for the safe delivery of a living child and for the "deliverance" of the mother.

13. Schrader was often vehement in her criticisms of other midwives, her criticisms tending to be rather more "destructive" than "constructive". There is not a single reference in the memoirs commending the techniques of other midwives, or involving the giving of advice or instruction. Certain midwives came in for special and frequent condemnation. While other midwives may well have been clumsy and inept, even "torturers" as Schrader refers to them, her comments might have been partly the result of competitiveness and professional jealousy, and as such not completely founded.

14. Leeuwarden is approximately 15 kilometers from Marrum, a considerable distance by the standards of the period.

15. Vrouw Schrader used instruments, usually a hook or crotchet (probably the most commonly used instrument in obstetric practice during this period), as a last resort when all other attempts to deliver had failed, and almost without exception when the child was already dead. Schrader used both the techniques of embriotomy and craniotomy. In most cases instrumental deliveries took place in the presence of a surgeon or man-midwife, who often assisted.

16. Schrader frequently refers to being present at confinements for one "etmaal", and so on. There is no equivalent word in English for this time period, which literally means 24 hours, a day and a night. When the expression occurs in the text, it has been translated as a "whole day".

17. Vrouw Schrader wrote this case up twice in her memoirs, but only once in her notebook. The duplication of the case here indicates that she sometimes re-wrote case histories.

18. Ameland is a large island off North Friesland. Schrader travelled there by boat, after a journey overland of approximately 14 kilometers from Hallum to the coast.

19. Schrader frequently practised "internal podalic version", a difficult manual technique which she was much experienced in, and usually successful in implementing. The manoeuvre consisted of "turning the birth to the feet", that is, of bringing the feet of the child to the orifice of the womb, and then pulling the child out by traction. This could be extremely effective in practised hands, unlike the

other manual techniques of labial stretching and cephalic version (converting malpresentations to head presentations). But it was by no means an easy technique, and probably could only be learned through repeated practice. Adrian Wilson, *Childbirth in Seventeenth- and Eighteenth-Century England*, 26-29.

20. The closure of the birth canal around the child's neck during delivery by podalic version was one of the dangers connected with this technique of delivery.
21. Vrouw Schrader moved from the village of Hallum to the town of Dokkum in December, 1695.
22. "Trekschuit" - a towboat or barge pulled by a horse.
23. The distance between Dokkum and Leeuwarden is well over twenty kilometers.
24. "Kraam" literally means "childbed". Schrader's use of the expression a "healthy childbed" is somewhat obscure, as she even describes protracted and dangerous deliveries, and cases where the child was dead or died during delivery, in this way. It seems most likely that she is referring to the woman's lying-in period and recovery following childbirth.
25. There were four gates to the town of Dokkum, the Aalsumerpoort, the Halvemaanspoort, the Hanspoort and the Woudpoort.
26. Sadly, Schrader gives little information concerning the ritual and ceremonial surrounding childbirth. Perhaps this is because these were difficult cases where much of the ceremonial had to be abandoned in the hope of saving the mother and child, and because Schrader herself was so dominant in the delivery scene. However, the attendance and assistance of women friends and neighbours seems to have been of some importance. For the ceremony surrounding childbirth, see, for example, Adrian Wilson, "Participant or patient? Seventeenth century childbirth from the mother's point of view", in: Roy Porter (ed.), *Patients and practitioners. Lay perceptions of medicine in pre-industrial society* (Cambridge: Cambridge University Press, 1986) 129-144.
27. Schrader often utilised the technique of placing the parturient woman "on her head" to turn the child or deliver it from behind. This technique, of "pitch-poling" the woman, was also recommended by the English obstetrician Willughby in cases where the child needed to be turned (podalic version). He described the technique, with the aid of a bolster, thus: "place a woman sitting on the bed, with a pillow on her lap, & her legs spread as wide, as she can conveniently, & place this bolster as nigh as may be to her knees. Then bring the woman [in labour], and cause her to kneel on this bolster, spreading abroad her knees; after this put her head down to the pillow lying in the woman's lap; then is she fitted for the turning of the child, or drawing it with the crotchett. When I use the word pitch-poling the woman, I mean to put her head down to the pillow as she kneeleth on the bolster." Percival Willughby, *Observations in Midwifery*, Sloane MS. 529, ff 1-19. Quoted in Adrian Wilson, *Childbirth in Seventeenth- and Eighteenth-Century England*, vol. II, Appendix B, 14.
28. During this period taken as a sign that the child was dead, especially when the navel string had ceased to pulsate.
29. Herbs were frequently employed during this period to ease or speed labour, to support the woman, stop bleeding and to expel dead births. Shorter cites the use by European midwives of ergot to strengthen uterine muscle contractions, roots of white lily, vermifuges and cinnamon sticks. Poppy, henbane, bryony root and pearlwort were also utilised to hasten labour. Edward Shorter, *A History of Women's Bodies*, 78; Mary Chamberlain, *Old Wives' Tales. Their history, remedies and spells* (London: Virago, 1981) 55. Schrader seemed to be particularly keen on

the technique of steaming the mother over a herbal bath to relax and soften the openings.

30. Leading as it did to complete obstruction, the arm presentation (transverse lie) was perhaps the most dreaded, and one which many midwives were not equipped to deal with. Many of the most gruesome acts of midwives were performed in cases of arm presentation. Some attempted to reduce the arm, either breaking it or failing to make it return; others cut the arm off, but the most usual procedure was to tug on the arm in an attempt to forcefully deliver the child. All these methods were both hopeless and dangerous. The only solution, and that normally adopted by Schrader, was to deliver by podalic version. Bringing down the feet caused the child to rotate and the arm or arms to be reduced automatically.

31. "Vlyger" - this phenomenon has been defined as a lump of meat which was driven from the body of the mother in a similar way to a miscarriage. It would appear to be similar to the "mole" described in *Aristotle's Works*, a "... great lump of hard flesh burdening the womb", formless, inanimate, and without human figure and affinity with the parent. *Aristotle's Works. The Works of the Famous Philosopher, containing his complete master-piece, and family physician, his experienced midwife* ... (author's own, London: The Booksellers, n.d., c. 1850 ed.) 79-80. It is also possible that a "vlyger" was a phantom which was believed, according to folk tradition, to fly into the woman's womb, the work of the devil or evil spirits.

32. The distance between Dokkum and Hantum is only five kilometers, but between Hantum and Bergum it is approximately twenty, a considerable distance for a midwife to travel to a delivery.

33. "Kop of" - literally "head off", a nickname with a rather obscure meaning - possibly someone who was not very bright, or someone small or with a small head!

34. During this period it was extremely difficult to tell whether or not the child still lived following a protracted or complicated labour, and this was of most relevance when a decision had to be reached over the delivery of a child with an instrument. The only certain signs were the putrid discharges and odours which indicated that the child was already rotten. If the fontanelle was soft and pulseless this was considered as a sign of death, or if the cord was delivered and had ceased to pulsate, or if the meconium was passed. Many midwives tested where an arm or foot presented by dipping it into cold water, believing that if the child still lived it would draw it in!

35. "Rinckelmantie" - a large basket.

36. Many midwives during this period allowed, or even recommended, the parturient woman to drink considerable quantities of alcohol - beer, wine or cordials. It was not unusual for the woman to be made so drunk that she was incapable of bearing down.

37. It is interesting to note that Vrouw Schrader carried her own set of instruments, and therefore could resort to instrumental deliveries without the presence of a man-midwife or surgeon.

38. Farrow - a litter of pigs.

39. Imagination was believed to act upon the developing foetus, and it was therefore important for the mother to avoid seeing, experiencing or thinking about anything that might mark the child. This included certain foods, ugly sights, animals and sudden frights. These things were blamed for any marks or deformities in the child. The birth of monsters was also attributed directly to God's will or the devil's doings.

40. This description sounds exaggerated, but fistulas and tears in the vaginal wall,

cervix and perineal tissues, and prolapsed uterus, all of whi-h would lead to extreme pain and difficulties in future deliveries, were common. The displacement of the womb downward, the "falling of the womb", sometimes through the vaginal opening, caused untold misery for women. See, for example, Edward Shorter, *A History of Women's Bodies*, 268-275.

41. See footnote 31 for an explanation of "vlygers". "Sugers" were apparently the same phenomena as "vlygers".

42. Caudle was a warm gruel heated with spice, sugar, and wine, used for invalids, but particularly associated with childbirth. The preparation of caudle played an important ceremonial role, and following the delivery, the custom was for the women of the neighbourhood to come to drink caudle in celebration of the birth.

43. A hundred guilders was an enormous sum of money at this time. The fee for a "top" midwife or obstetrician for an attendance of several weeks at a delivery of a very wealthy family would perhaps be as much as fifty guilders, half the amount mentioned by Schrader.

44. The problem of a contracted pelvis, often the result of rickets, was one frequently encountered by midwives and male obstetric attendants. When the pelvic bones were not large enough to accommodate the child's head this led to enormous difficulties in childbirth. If the woman was unable to deliver spontaneously or by version, the only solution, before the widespread introduction of caesarean section, was some kind of mutilating operation on the child, if the woman was not to die undelivered.

45. Cataplasm - a poultice or soft external application.

46. Kuikhoorn is approximately ten kilometers from Dokkum.

47. A great many midwives around this time "broke the waters" with a fingernail, scissors, razor or any other sharp object that they had to hand as a matter of course once labour had begun. This could be said to be part of the practice of "meddlesome midwifery", and an attempt to speed up the birth process. Schrader seems to have practised this technique, which could endanger the child and cause difficulties in the delivery, only rarely, and she berated other midwives for their haste in rupturing the "sack".

48. A small coin, approximately 1.5 cm in diameter.

49. A coin, approximately 3 cm in diameter.

50. Presumably a case of hydrocephalus.

51. "Ramsnoes" - nose of a ram.

52. "Geneva" - Dutch gin.

53. Presumably a case of spina bifida.

54. There are no extracts in the notebook for case numbers 2809 to 2823.

SELECT BIBLIOGRAPHY

The Dutch edition of Vrouw Schrader's notebook appeared in 1984:
M.J. van Lieburg (ed.), *C.G. Schraders Memoryboeck van de Vrouwens. Het notitieboek van een Friese vroedvrouw 1693-1745. Met een verloskundig commentaar van Prof.Dr. G.J. Kloosterman*, Amsterdam: Editions Rodopi, 1984 (1st and 2nd editions) and 1985 (3rd edition).

Vrouw Schrader and her notebook:

M.J. Elzinga, "Catharina Geertruid Schraders 1655-1745", *It Beaken* 16 (1954) 192-196.

W.Th.M. Frijhoff, "Vrouw Schraders beroepsjournaal: overwegingen bij een publikatie over arbeidspraktijk in het verleden", *Tijdschr. Gesch. Geneesk. Natuurwet. Wisk. Techn.* 8 (1985) 27-38.

A. Geyl, "Catharina Geetruyd Schrader. Investigatrice du caractère anatomique de la placenta praevia", *Janus* 1 (1896-1897) 537-540.

Chr. van Kammen, *C.G. Schraders Memorijboeck van de vrouwens. Dagboek van verlossingen te Dokkum 1693-1745*, Dokkum: Gemeentebestuur, 1958 (stencilled edition).

B.W.Th. Nuyens, "Het dagboek van Vrouw Schraders. Een bijdrage tot de geschiedenis der verloskunde in de 17de en 18e eeuw", *Ned. Tijdschr. Geneesk.* 70 (1926) II, 1790-1791.

Obstetrics in The Netherlands:

A.C. Drogendijk, *De verloskundige voorziening in Dordrecht van ca. 1500 tot heden*, Amsterdam: H.J. Paris, 1935.

A.J. van Reeuwijk, *Vroedkunde en vroedvrouwen in de Nederlanden in de 17e en 18e eeuw*, n.p. 1941.

General literature on obstetrics and midwifery:

J.H. Aveling, *English Midwives*, London: J. & A. Churchill, 1872, reprinted New York: AMS Press, 1977.

Jane B. Donegan, *Women & Men Midwives. Medicine, Morality, and Misogyny in Early America*, Westport, Conn. and London: Greenwood Press, 1978.

Jean Donnison, *Midwives and Medical Men. A History of Inter-Professional Rivalries and Women's Rights*, New York: Schocken, 1977.

Audrey Eccles, *Obstetrics and Gynaecology in Tudor and Stuart England*, London: Croom Helm, 1982.

Mireille Laget, "Childbirth in Seventeenth- and Eighteenth-Century France: Obstetrical Practices and Collective Attitudes", in: Robert Forster and Orest Ranum (eds.), *Medicine and Society in France. Selections from the Annales*, vol. 6 (Baltimore: Johns Hopkins University Press, 1980) 137-176.

Judith Walzer Leavitt, *Brought to Bed. Childbearing in America 1750 to 1950*, New York and Oxford: Oxford University Press, 1986.

Judith Walzer Leavitt (ed.), *Women and Health in America*, Madison, Wisconsin: University of Wisconsin Press, 1984.

Judy Barrett Litoff, *The American midwife debate. A sourcebook on its modern origins*, Westport, Conn. and London: Greenwood Press, 1986.

Judy Barrett Litoff, *American Midwives 1860 to the Present*, Westport, Conn. and London: Greenwood Press, 1978.

Irvine Loudon, "Deaths in childbed from the eighteenth century to 1935" *Medical History* 30 (1986) 1-41.

Catherine M. Scholten, *Childbearing in American Society, 1650-1850*, ed. by Lynne Withey, New York and London: New York University Press, 1985.

Edward Shorter, *A History of Women's Bodies*, New York, Basic Books, 1982.

Herbert R. Spencer, *The History of British Midwifery From 1650 to 1800*, London: John Bale, Sons & Danielsson, 1927; reprinted AMS Press: New York, 1978.

Richard W. and Dorothy C. Wertz, *Lying-In. A History of Childbirth in America*, New York: Schocken, 1979.

Adrian Wilson, *Childbirth in Seventeenth- and Eighteenth-Century England* (unpublished PhD thesis), University of Sussex, 1982.

Adrian Wilson, "Participant or patient? Seventeenth century childbirth from the mother's point of view", in: Roy Porter (ed.), *Patients and practitioners. Lay perceptions of medicine in pre-industrial society* (Cambridge: Cambridge University Press, 1986) 129-144.

Adrian Wilson, *A Safe Deliverance: ritual and conflict in English childbirth, 1600-1750*, Cambridge: Cambridge University Press, forthcoming 1988.

CONTRIBUTORS

Kloosterman, G.J., Emeritus Professor of Obstetrics and Gynaecology of the University of Amsterdam.

Lieburg, F.A. van, Student of History, Erasmus University Rotterdam.

Lieburg, M.J. van, Professor of Medical History of the Free University Amsterdam and the Erasmus University Rotterdam.

Marland, Hilary, Research Officer, Free University Amsterdam and Erasmus University Rotterdam.

CPSIA information can be obtained at www.ICGtesting.com
Printed in the USA
BVOW040554230513

321449BV00001B/6/A